VACCINE SCIENCE REVISITED

Are Childhood Immunizations As Safe As Claimed?

JAMES&LANCE
MORCAN

VACCINE SCIENCE REVISITED: Are Childhood Immunizations As Safe As Claimed?

Published by:
Sterling Gate Books
28 St. Heliers Place,
Papamoa 3118,
Bay of Plenty,
New Zealand
sterlinggatebooks@gmail.com

National Library of New Zealand publication data:
Morcan, James 1978-
Morcan, Lance 1948-
Title: VACCINE SCIENCE REVISITED: Are Childhood Immunizations As Safe As Claimed?
Edition: First ed.
Format: Paperback
Publisher: Sterling Gate Books
ISBN: 978-0-473-52159-2

TABLE OF CONTENTS

"I think of the need for more wisdom in the world, to deal with the knowledge that we have. At one time we had wisdom, but little knowledge. Now we have a great deal of knowledge, but do we have enough wisdom to deal with that knowledge?"

~ Jonas Salk

ACKNOWLEDGEMENTS

Elísabet (Lisa) Norris, Medical Laboratory Scientist: For carefully reading this manuscript at various stages over the years and seeing potential in our early, raw drafts. For patiently advising us on how to improve it again and again. And also for sharing insider tales of what goes on in medical labs and public healthcare facilities. We cannot thank you enough, Lisa!

Dr. Stephen Martino, M.D.: For sharing details about the field of neurology and also offering personal insights as a father who oversaw and observed vaccination of his own children.

Denis Toovey, Clinical Pharmacist and author of *Better Health for You:* For collaborating with us on our previous medical non-fiction book, which helped prepare us to put together the pieces of this healthcare jigsaw.

Dr. Kevin Coleman: For alerting us to anomalies in vaccine research and answering numerous scientific questions over the years. Also for sharing personal experiences of administering vaccines on various continents during his professional medical career.

Sigríður Ó. Einarsdóttir, Registered Nurse: For reading the manuscript and giving honest feedback.

Leticia Martinez: For encouragement and being a positive force.

Tammi Stefano: For setting an example of how to be courageous and stand up for the truth.

Lastly, we'd like to thank the more than 13,000 members of *Underground Knowledge,* the global discussion group we founded on Goodreads. Especially the doctors, scientists, nurses and parents who bravely shared their opinions about vaccines in a public forum.

FOREWORD

Back when I was a student in the laboratory science program at Weber State University, Utah, I developed a fascination for microbial life. Vaccine science was a part of the curriculum, but the emphasis, ahead of all else, was on the greatness of the invention of vaccines and their revolutionary ability to ward off sickness. Vaccines were then, and still are, considered a lifesaving technology. Said to be so crucial to our health that every child should receive the official immunization schedule, which in some countries is now mandatory by law.

During my student days, there was never any opportunity for discussion relating to potential downsides to the vaccination process and we were even encouraged, albeit subtly, to debunk anyone who dared question the safety of the many vaccines in circulation.

What we didn't learn as students, and something you don't commonly hear about when being vaccinated, is what a vaccine's ingredients or contaminants are (not to mention their potential side effects).

The microbial, or bacteriological, realm inside us always continued to intrigue me. Even after completing my formal studies at university and commencing work as a medical laboratory scientist, I conducted personal research into this unique world in my downtime. It wasn't until more recent years however, that I came across research papers and articles on vaccines that led me to develop some reservations in regards to their manufacture. This was literally the first time, after many years of studying medicine and working in the healthcare sector, that vaccines became a concern to me.

Having two teenage kids who are both fully vaccinated, healthy and without allergies or disabilities of any kind, I can't say my concern over vaccines and their side effects related to me personally. Yet having worked at a medical clinic for many years it was not lost on me how often children were falling ill and being diagnosed with some type of disease.

1

As I started to research further, I began to wonder whether there could be a valid correlation between vaccines and at least some of these diagnosed childhood diseases.

Trying to find such a correlation turned out to be more difficult than expected. Vaccine research is often convoluted or else too narrowly focused. I also came to realize how difficult it is to distinguish between legitimate research and biased research. It became clear to me that many of the research papers I was studying were misrepresenting true observations.

I have great respect for researchers and the passion they put into their work. The papers they publish are often ground-breaking and fascinating. Unfortunately though, science has its own version of *fake news*.

This was highlighted in shocking fashion in October of 2018 when the world's news media reported that three academics—Dr. Peter Boghossian, Helen Pluckrose and Dr. James Lindsay—had cleverly exposed the weaknesses of scientific journals. In order to prove a point about shoddy research standards, they made up research and created their own data to fit a pre-conceived conclusion and sent these papers off to peer-reviewed journals. Some of these papers made it through peer review and were actually published.

That and other examples of serious flaws in the field of scientific research have forced me to view other scientists' work with a more critical eye.

In the first part of this book, authors James and Lance Morcan put vaccine ingredients under the microscope one at a time and explain their effects on cells within the human body. This is a journey like no other. The reader is given an insight into how the vaccine ingredients themselves impact our cells and what happens to us when our cells are exposed to them.

The second part of this book inspects the various illnesses associated with the ingredients found in childhood vaccines. At times the dangers seem so obvious you start wondering why it isn't clear to everyone.

Vaccine Science Revisited opens your eyes to so much more than just vaccines. It makes the reader realize how affected we are by our environment in general. And all of a sudden, all the various disorders humankind puts up with start making more sense. We are shown how multitudes of factors play their part and how these make it so difficult for medical professionals to determine a specific cause for an illness. Because most likely, there isn't a specific cause, but an accumulation of multiple causes.

James and Lance have done an extraordinary job digging through paper after paper in order to find the most authentic and reliable studies to include in this book. It's extremely rare to find a book that covers vaccines in such a scientifically pure manner. In other words, the data is presented in its raw state so nothing should cloud the reader's judgement or taint the research.

Again though, it's also nearly impossible to distinguish between fake data and true data. So in the end, it's difficult to know which scientific authors or papers to trust when researching immunization studies. To combat this, James and Lance have searched for consistency using papers from multiple authors in order to uncover true or accurate data.

Although the human body can't be dissected into fragments and problems cannot usually be pinpointed to specific locations, this book also does a great job at explaining how various vaccine ingredients can impact our cells.

Focusing on our cellular levels is so important in this field of research because cells cover our entire body. So rather than narrowing our perspective solely to damage within one location of the body, we obtain a broader, more holistic view by studying the influence of vaccine ingredients on cells. It becomes clear when reading this book that what happens in one part of the body has consequences on other parts of the body as well.

Cells that comprise the human body are extremely intricate, yet observable. Using the information of some of the cellular functions mentioned in this book, you can clearly imagine certain mechanisms within a cell and how each and every part (of a cell) has a job to do.

One of my favorite revelations in this book is the importance of the cell membrane and how it regulates exactly what enters and leaves the cell. The authors opened my mind to possibilities I hadn't ever fully considered. One good example being that the cell membrane doesn't just regulate the entrance to the cell, it also controls what happens within the cell.

Substances contained in vaccines are able to alter or destroy membranes, which influences the mechanisms and duties they perform within the cell. What's most fascinating about this, if you take a deeper look at cellular function and consider everything within the cell as merely a factory with workers, is each cell needs commands in order to know what to do. Everything is on standby until a command is given.

If you asked yourself where these commands are coming from, the answer surely must be: from outside the cell. If that's the case, then ask yourself: what's the most important aspect of this whole process?

Could it possibly be the membrane? The membrane decides what messages to allow in and which ones to block. Those it allows in carry the commands for the cellular components to perform. Those (messages) it blocks are commands the cellular components won't perform. When the membrane malfunctions, the components can't perform properly. This goes for the production of DNA as well because DNA production is also a cellular function.

Keeping all that in mind, this book illustrates the magic of our body's ability to regulate itself and how outside influences can affect us. We are reminded we must take good care of these cellular mechanisms and keep our cellular membranes intact. We need them in order to maintain and control proper cellular functions, which in turn is what keeps us healthy.

Therefore, to fully understand the impact vaccines have on our bodies requires a much broader investigation than even most of my scientific colleagues would assume necessary.

Although this book is essentially about vaccine ingredients and their effects, what's great is all the information shared also provides an insight into how our environment in general can alter us. It's skilfully constructed to cater equally for those who are strong believers in mainstream science and those who are focused more on *rogue scientists*. Since the facts are presented in their purest form, people of all beliefs can use the material in this book to further their understanding of this contentious medical subject.

In my opinion, James and Lance Morcan have pulled off an almost impossible task. To wrangle with the vast amounts of medical data and not only make sense of it, but satisfactorily explain it all to the layman while providing sufficient sources and references to satisfy readers with medical degrees, is a major intellectual achievement.

I strongly urge anybody, regardless of academic standing or lack thereof, to read this book and familiarize themselves with the concepts presented in it. *Vaccine Science Revisited: Are Childhood Immunizations As Safe As Claimed?* will be with me as a constant reference guide and a reminder that I, too, have control over what happens to my cells.

Elísabet Norris (Medical Laboratory Scientist, B.S.)

INTRODUCTION

Remember those infamous pox parties where parents deliberately exposed children to diseases such as the flu virus, measles and chickenpox? They were especially popular in the United States and in Britain at one stage—the idea being that children build immunity after being exposed to an infectious disease like chickenpox, which is more dangerous to adults than children. That was back in the day, before vaccinations were available, although it seems such activities persist to the present day in some quarters if mainstream media reports are accurate.

We certainly aren't advocating parents arrange pox parties to immunize their children. However, we mention those parties as they represent a schism that still exists to a degree in regards to approaches to guard against the wrath of infectious diseases.

Paradoxical as it may sound, it has traditionally been considered a good thing when a child gets sick with certain infectious diseases like chicken pox early in life. The idea being that children develop a long-term immunity from exposure to such diseases.

Of course, isolated experiences of children growing up to become healthy adults after early exposure like this does not take away the very real threats diseases pose to children, especially those in poverty-stricken areas of our fragile planet. There's a multitude of frightening accounts of deformities, suffering and death resulting from some of these diseases. It is therefore highly commendable that scientists and others strive to develop ways to prevent children from succumbing to disease and falling ill.

Vaccine Science Revisited, or at least the research process that led to its creation, has been about half a century in the making. As the following shows, our investigation into vaccines, child vaccines in particular, began by mere happenstance.

The older one of us (Lance) started actively researching child vaccines as a young newspaper and broadcasting journalist in the late 1960s and early 1970s. This entailed visiting hospitals and medical clinics in New Zealand and Australia, and interviewing doctors and nurses as well as parents.

Scientific research into vaccines was fairly new back then and much has changed since those *early times*. What's interesting is the immunization schedule of recommended vaccines was considerably less then than the amount of vaccines that are recommended, *or in some cases are mandatory,* today.

Over the decades, we have monitored from afar the sciences that relate to vaccines. A sometimes overwhelming task that included reading various books by scientists, following news stories written by other investigative journalists on vaccines, and talking to laboratory technicians, doctors and nurses about the immunization process.

In more recent years we made several attempts to begin writing this book. However, we always found the research required was simply too exhaustive and kept putting it aside to work on other (less intellectually demanding) book and film projects.

In 2015, we published a book called *Medical Industrial Complex,* which aimed to expose the financial corruption and conflicts of interest that exist in modern medicine. Doing research for that particular book saw us not only interviewing doctors, nurses and other medical professionals once more, but also collaborating with a veteran pharmacist. It opened our eyes to some alarming practices within modern medicine that we hadn't previously considered. Cozy relationships between supposedly independent and unbiased divisions of the healthcare sector being one of those, and the shutting down of potentially worthy medical debates because of financial interests, academic rigidity or even political correctness being another.

Although we briefly touched on vaccines in that book, it was admittedly more of a cursory overview. We still did not feel sufficiently knowledgeable or well-researched to accurately assess the science behind the modern immunization process. Nor had we, at that stage, a clear picture of the dramatic and often torturous early history of vaccinations. A history which makes for compelling reading and which we address in the first few chapters of this book.

Around the same time we started a global discussion group called *Underground Knowledge* on Goodreads—the popular, Amazon-owned, social media site for book readers. It soon became (and continues to be) an excellent forum for public debate on vaccinations and medicine in general, attracting concerned parents and social activists as well as doctors, scientists and other medical professionals with firsthand experience in either administering vaccines or working with them in laboratories.

We ran a group poll asking members, Do you believe child immunizations/vaccines are for the most part extremely safe as per official statements from mainstream medicine and Big Pharma? The poll received 501 total votes of which 281 (56.1%) voted Yes. However, 220 voted either No or Unsure. The numbers of poll respondents in doubt, combined with certain comments made by medical practitioners, finally inspired us enough to attempt to drill down to deeper levels of medical research papers, do the hard yards and write the book you are reading now.

At first, we felt more like fence-sitters as we were simply observing all sides and listening to the various arguments. We also knew we wouldn't be able to make up our own minds simply by reading other people's statements. We had to attain a stronger comprehension of the medical sciences at hand to gain an educated and informed understanding of vaccines.

A lifetime's interest in health combined with our previous investigations into the medical sector, or sectors, had taught us that nature often finds ways to take care of itself, the human body included. We realized early on in our research there was a real concern about introducing the body to toxins it has never had to deal with before. Toxins that enter the body unnaturally and bypass our natural defense system.

It became apparent to us the body reacts differently to these toxins depending on the route of entry. This adds a further complexity to the whole vaccination issue. A complexity that would present challenges for us when sifting through study designs while gathering appropriate information on vaccine ingredients.

Since these vaccines are approved and deemed safe, we had to consider that perhaps the amount of toxins (in vaccines) are small enough that our body can accommodate and process them without a problem. After all, it is a part of our body armor's design to filter out and eliminate toxins. This works well for healthy individuals, but we soon realized that, unfortunately, in today's society there are countless children with weakened immune systems whose protective armor is not as strong.

Although these children are in minority, we feel strongly they should not be tossed to the wayside and ignored.

If vaccines really are unsafe for children with permanently weakened immune systems, they could also be unsafe or risky for the majority of children whenever their usually healthy immune systems are temporarily in a weakened condition for whatever reason.

On that note, after we started reading the package inserts for each vaccine, we realized that all the inserts come with warnings on who should *not* be given vaccines. Check these package inserts out. They make for very interesting reading.

After talking to many parents who have taken their children in for immunizations, it appears the information given to them about the shots is limited to which diseases the shots are for. Other than that, the parents are essentially left in the dark.

When we approached doctors and nurses about this issue, many said they don't have time to read all the package inserts, relying instead on what they are being told by "the experts" supplying the product. This motivated us to include them (medical professionals) in our long list of people this book is written for as we realized they often have little background knowledge on vaccine science. Which meant we had to make it *sciencey* enough to be taken seriously by them.

We were under no illusions doctors, nurses, surgeons and other medical professionals would require much convincing because many we approached indicated they, and they alone, had science on their side. We reached this inescapable conclusion because they told us to "believe in the science" or "just read the medical journals." In fact, we lost count how many of these professionals recited those phrases, oftentimes verbatim!

Unfortunately, such comments usually came without any further explanation. It was as if these medical professionals thought those comments spoke for themselves as proof that vaccines are always completely safe and beneficial—and should never be questioned, apparently.

It's an unfortunate truth that modern science, like mainstream medicine, has been shown to be corrupt at times, or unconsciously biased at other times, and is often fallible. Make no mistake, we greatly respect scientific and mainstream medical journals as evidenced by the fact that about 90% of this book is simply references to, or reports and reviews of, official medical papers prepared by scientists. *However,* our caveat is that the facts and observations presented in such documents must be unbiased and untainted by academic dogma, pursuit of fame and profit, or any of the other failings that jeopardize medical research.

We are aware some of our findings will upset those who are for vaccines, and some definitely won't be popular with those against them. It wasn't our goal to prove either *side* right or wrong, but to clarify where their arguments originate from and to revisit those origins, leaving the science to do the talking. We honestly had no idea where our research and reviews of medical papers would take us, and we were ready to accept the facts as long as they were appropriately presented.

Little did we know how difficult it would be to source scientific and medical research that could be trusted as containing untainted or unbiased data. We soon found ourselves buried in research and began questioning our ability to tackle this monster of a subject. Conservatively, we would have read or at least skimmed more than a thousand research documents and papers. It was so overwhelming we were forced to rethink our strategy.

We realized we needed to be pickier about the papers we chose to investigate, and so we did exactly that. We also brought together a team of medical advisors, including a doctor, lab scientists and other healthcare practitioners, who, between them, helped us develop the right approach to researching this complex field.

This turned out to the best decision we made with this book. Our search through the research paper pile no longer seemed impossible as we finally had clear guidelines to work to. And so we started focusing on such things as who the authors of the studies were, where the studies were performed, how large the population sample was, who was included in the study, and the design of each study. It took us a while, but we were able to discard most studies after developing a list of qualifying criteria studies needed to pass if they were to be considered.

Being able to work with a team of people who know how to read research papers, and bounce questions off them, was like a breath of fresh air.

One good piece of advice we received from our medical advisory team was that after we found any research papers that met the qualifying criteria, we couldn't just read the abstract or the conclusion. This, our experts informed us, was the problem for many health professionals. They simply don't have the time to read the research, so they make do with the abstract or sometimes just the study's conclusion. This forced us to read through entire research papers.

Throughout our epic dive into the world of research papers, we realized that when it came to researching vaccines and their ingredients, many of them do not have adequate research data available. In order to find out the impact these ingredients or contaminants have, we found ourselves frequently forced to lean on research *unrelated to* vaccines or lean on research with a bias to fit either the hypothesis or the funding entity's interest.

It was at times very difficult, sometimes even impossible, to find articles by independent researchers accepted by the mainstream scientific community. Our feelings were supported by others in the scientific field as well.

An article from granbydrummer.com states:

> *"One reason this topic is so controversial is because long-term studies by independent organizations have not been allowed in the United States. Only limited independent information is available to the public and politicians. This contradicts scientific research methods in the U.S.A."* [1]

Another important point regarding research papers is the fact that it is very difficult for people in general, but especially those *outside* the scientific community, to know which sets of data are reliable.

In an article by Richard Horton (*FMedSci*), Editor-in-Chief of *The Lancet,* he states:

> *"The case against science is straightforward: much of the scientific literature, perhaps half, may simply be untrue. Afflicted by studies with small sample sizes, tiny effects, invalid exploratory analyses, and flagrant conflicts of interest, together with an obsession for pursuing fashionable trends of dubious importance, science has taken a turn towards darkness. As one participant put it, 'poor methods get results.'"* [2]

It is very concerning for us to read such an article in a prestigious, peer-reviewed, medical journal like *The Lancet*. Horton's concern doesn't stop there.

Regarding researchers he says that in their:

> "...*quest for telling a compelling story, scientists too often sculpt data to fit their preferred theory of the world. Or they retrofit hypotheses to fit their data.*" [3]

His concern isn't just aimed at the researchers, either. He feels journal editors can be just as shady in their actions, and there is an "unhealthy competition" taking place in trying to get papers published in the more prominent journals.

Horton says that their:

> "... *love of 'significance' pollutes the literature with many a statistical fairy-tale. We reject important confirmations.*" [4]

It seems it isn't just the researchers and journal editors who are desperate for favorable research. Universities are also seeking "money and talent."

Sadly, and somewhat surprisingly, in his conclusion of the aforementioned article where Horton summarizes his attendance at a symposium on the reproducibility and reliability of biomedical research, he says they could not think of a solution to this problem:

> "*The bad news is that nobody is ready to take the first step to clean up the system.*" [5]

In writing this book, we tried to be as diverse in our research as possible so as not to bias the reader. That said, we do of course have our own thoughts on vaccines, which are occasionally reflected in (fairly brief) commentaries scattered throughout the book. These are not meant to bias the facts presented, merely to share with you our thoughts.

Please note the word *Revisited* in this book's main title *Vaccine Science Revisited*. It refers to a new inspection of what the science actually says about vaccines and vaccinations.

We are aware many members of the general public and, especially, the scientific community believe any debate over vaccine effectiveness, or how safe vaccines are, should have ended long ago, and that "science has already conclusively spoken." We beg to differ, and we believe you will, too, once you read this book and consider the almost infinite number of murky, gray areas exposed by the vast amount of research out there. Too much has been assumed and misunderstood—on all sides.

It's definitely time for society to revisit the subject of vaccines and vaccine safety, especially where our children are concerned, and open up the scientific debate once more.

Keep in mind, however, the debate we are primarily focused on is not whether or not we should vaccinate/immunize our children. Rather, as this book's subtitle suggests, we are focused on whether childhood vaccines are as safe as claimed. For it is, after all, possible to be extremely pro-vaccines yet still wonder if they can *and should* be made safer. Likewise, it is also possible to be very pro science and anti-pseudoscience yet still question vaccine safety claims or else demand more effective safety protocols.

So, the aforementioned doctors and other medical professionals who dismissively replied to all our questions with "Believe in the science" or "Just read the medical journals" will be pleased to know we have done exactly that—and only that. We trust you'll appreciate how this book avoids all rumor, conjecture, conspiracy theories and anecdotal evidence, and steadfastly focuses on what the latest medical and scientific research *actually says* about vaccines.

Even if you are anti-vaccines, or else highly-skeptical of their safety, remember that if any of the most controversial theories are true then it must be possible for science to prove it. Eventually, any harmful vaccine ingredients will be proven to be just that. That's why we have excluded all theories and focused on facts contained in the best research data available.

Beyond all the controversy, naivety, paranoia, academic rigidity and Pollyannaish trust in governments and multinational pharmaceutical corporations, what does the most reliable and unbiased science actually reveal about vaccines?

Read on to find out. And no matter your level of education or experience—whether you are a doctor, layman, scientist, nurse, med student or new parent—be prepared to be surprised by much of the medical research findings.

James & Lance Morcan

Introduction:
1 Granby Drummer. (2018, March 1). *TIOSN presents: Soil, plant and human health effects of glyphosate*. Retrieved from www.granbydrummy.com/2018/03/tison-presents-soil-plant-and-human-healtheffects-of-glyphosate/
[2] Horton, R. (2015). Offline: What is medicine's 5 sigma? *The Lancet*, 385(9976), p1380
[3] Ibid.
[4] Ibid.
[5] Ibid.

PART ONE

Vaccine ingredients up close

CHAPTER 1

Force of nature

*"All living things contain a measure of
madness that moves them in strange, sometimes
inexplicable ways. This madness can be saving;
it is part and parcel of the ability to adapt.
Without it, no species would survive."*

~Yann Martel (Life of Pi)

On June 27th, 1833, a 21-year-old man suffered from severe head and back pain. One day later, he was still in great pain and red spots covered his body and face. Smallpox.

By morning, Surgeon Henry George[1] had come to see him. The surgeon wrote in his notebook:

*"His mind was wandering; his limbs and voice tremulous;
his tongue dry, and covered with a brownish-red crust
[...]."* [2]

The man's face was completely swollen from pustules. Surgeon George fed him beef-tea and arrow-root and gave him medication. This helped the young man sleep for a few hours during the night.

The morning after, the swelling was worse and the pustules had merged together and blanketed his face. By July 1st, five days after the illness started, his entire body had turned a bluish-gray color. The pustules covering his body were completely confluent. Calamine, which was often used to reduce smallpox scarring, was applied to his body.

His seizures were so intense that it took five people to hold him down. The seizures continued throughout his illness. By July 9th, nearly two weeks since he became sick, Surgeon George described the young man as:

"[…] the most horrid spectacle that can be imagined; lies, and while lying, trembles from head to foot; his countenance suspiciously wild, and expressive of the darkest intentions; […]."[3]

From other accounts of what smallpox does to a person, we can assume the pain was unbearable. Infected skin cells shedding as the virus struggled for survival. With the skin peeling off, the virus escaped to re-enter the body via such means as saliva. Once in the saliva, the germ infected the digestive system, giving it access to all organs.

The pustules grew to the size of boils, and any physical touch excruciating. The slightest movement would have felt like the skin being torn off. Still, through all this, the young man stayed fully alert.

Surgeon George continued to explain how a couple of days later, the outer layer of skin had completely detached itself from the rest of his face. Although the surgeon did not describe his patient being any pain, we cannot help but wonder how painful the separation of skin from his face must have been. The nerves would have been exposed without a layer of protection.

Surgeon George described infections under both big toes and in one of the heels. The infections oozed a rancid bloody discharge. The smell, he described as "dreadful."

Three weeks later, on August 30th, the surgeon notes that his patient had:

"[…] violent flushing of the face; he is now pale, cold, a degree of stupor hanging over him; very dilated pupil; cannot tell the hour, and seems unconscious of your presence […] he does not now walk erect; in moving, his motions are very hurried, and his body considerably bent."[4]

The surgeon continues to treat him with medication and wine. His last notes end on September 2nd with the patient more pleasant and reading the newspaper. The illness had consumed two full months of his life. He had survived the smallpox attack. He would live the rest of his life with major scarring to his face and body.

Stories of severe illnesses are not uncommon throughout our human history. Neither are the stories of humans' innate desire for survival. We fight to prevent diseases and we fight to heal in the aftermath.

Desperate measures have been the groundwork for development of various techniques to ward off and to treat diseases. Even before our understanding of pathogens, or disease-causing germs, we were hard at work battling them. Often alchemy and superstitious practices became the main focus.

One such technique was described by a Chinese talisman, referred to in the book *Chu yu shih-san kho*[5], on how to exorcize the smallpox out of a child:

> *"[…] write the magic character on paper with red cinnabar ink, burn it to ashes, and have the child take them in liquid."*[6]

Later on, these practices became more medicine-oriented. An example of such a source that explains various variolation, or inoculation techniques is *I tsung chin chien* (*The Golden Mirror of Medicine*). This is a collection of all available treatises, gathered together in 1739 by the Imperial College of Physicians in Peking. This collection contained four ways to prevent smallpox—as listed here:

> *"Aqueous inoculum method (shui miao fa). Allow a moistened plug of cotton-wool to imbibe an aqueous extract of a number of pulverised scabs (chia), and insert it into a nostril of the child to be inoculated.*
>
> *"Dry inoculum method (han miao fa). Use slowly dried scabs, grind them into a fine powder, and blow it into the child's nostrils by a suitable tube of silver.*
>
> *"Smallpox-garment method (tou i fa). Wrap the child or the patient in a garment which has been worn by a smallpox sufferer during the illness.*
>
> *"Smallpox lymph method (tou chiang fa). Impregnate a plug of cotton-wool with lymph from the perfectly matured pustules of a smallpox patient, and insert this into the nostril of the child to be inoculated."*[7]

The Chinese knew how virulent the virus being used for the inoculum was. This was very important as it dictated its safety and efficacy. A man by the name of Yü Thien-chhih[8] explained how inoculates were only collected from patients with mild symptoms. They collected only from patients who had a mild strain of the virus. Any other more virulent or epidemic-type strains were considered too dangerous to use and would kill people, rather than immunize them.

In addition to the potency factor of various strains, Yü Thien-chhih mentions a monetary benefit to inoculation in a collection called *Sha tou chi chieh* from 1727:

> *"[...] you have to pay two or three pieces of gold for enough to inoculate one person. Physicians who want to make some profit pass it through the children of their own relatives. [...] Others eager for money steal away the scabs from [severe] smallpox cases and use the material directly. It is called pai miao (ruined inoculum). In such cases there will be 15 deaths in 100 patients."*[9]

Tibetans have been performing inoculations since ancient times as well. Their method was to dip multiple needles into a solution containing the virus and dried crusts. Using the dipped needles, they would prick the arm of the individual being immunized.

Needle-pricks around the world

Inoculations seemed to be happening across borders worldwide. Turkey was known for its success with inoculations. While staying in Turkey's (then) capital Constantinople, in December, 1713, the renowned Fellow of London's Royal Society, Mr. Emanuel Timonius, wrote a letter about this practice and how smallpox inoculations have already been in use for 40 years in Turkey.

During these inoculations, not a single person had died. In his letter, Mr. Timonius describes the procedure:

> *"[...] Needle prick the Tubercles [...] press out the Matter coming from them into some convenient vessel of Glass [...] wash and clean the Vessel first with warm Water: A convenient quantity of this Matter being thus collected, is to be Stop'd close, and kept warm in the Bosom of the Person that carries it, and, as Soon as may be, brought to the place of expecting future Patient."*[10]

He continued explaining that after the patient received the inoculant:

"[...] the Operator is to make several little Wounds with a Needle, in one, two or more places of the Skin, till some drops of Blood follow, and immediately drop out some drops of the Matter in the Glass, and mix it well with the Blood issuing out [...]."[11]

In 1717, while residing in Turkey, Lady Mary Wortley, an English aristocrat, writer and wife of the British ambassador in Turkey, wrote letters encouraging the methods to be used in England. She had herself been sick with smallpox, and it left her face quite scarred. She didn't want that for her five-year-old son, and requested Charles Maitland, the embassy surgeon at the time, to inoculate him.

When they returned to England, Maitland received a royal license to conduct an experiment on death row prisoners.[12] So, in 1721, Charles Maitland, Dr. Richard Mead, Sir Hans

Sloane and Dr. John George Steigerthal performed an experiment at Newgate Prison[13] in London.[14]

After the prisoners were inoculated, they were sent to Hertford. There was a smallpox epidemic there at the time.[15] None of the prisoners got sick with smallpox. All the prisoners in the experiment survived and were excused of their crimes in return for participating in the experiment.

Princess Caroline of Great Britain was not quite ready to inoculate her own children, even after the successful experimentation on the prisoners. In order to confirm its success, she had six orphans inoculated. None of the orphans became sick with smallpox when exposed. The princess now felt comfortable enough to inoculate her own children.

Chapter 1: Force of nature

[1] Google. (2018, December 16). Henry George Surgeon, Surgeon Extraordinaire to H.R.H. the Duke of Gloucester. Retrieved from www.google.com/search?hl=en&biw=664&bih=643&tbm=bks&ei=pFkWXK6X OqWJ0gLuwpHIBA&q=Henry+George+Surgeon%2C+Surgeon+Extraordinary +to+H.+R.+H.+the+Duke+of+Gloucester&oq=Henry+George+Surgeon%2C +Surgeon+Extraordinary+to+H.+R.+H.+the+Duke+of+Gloucester&gs_l=psy-ab.3...90762.94495.0.94914.13.13.0.0.0.0.126.1269.3j9.12.0....0...1c.1.64.psy-ab..1.0.0....0.1seS-AoRibc

[2] Henry, George. (1833). *A Compendious History of Small-pox* (pp. 103-104). London: Idotson and Palmer, Churchill.

[3] Ibid. (p. 107).

[4] Ibid. (p. 112).

[5] "The thirteen departments of apotropaic medicine", which was written sometime after 1456 AD. This is not the oldest source of variolation. The first account of variolation mentioned, is rumored to be in Ishino, which is a collection of Chinese medical sources from 982 AD.

[6] Needham, J., Gwei-Djen, L. and Sivin, N. (2004). *Science and Civilisation in China, Vol 6-6 Biology and Biological Technology Medicine* (p. 160). United Kingdom: Cambridge University Press,

[7] Ibid. (pp. 141-142).

[8] According to Joseph Needham In *Science and Civilsation in China, Vol 6-6 Biology and Biological Technology Medicine* Yu was also "called the 'strange man' who brought the inoculation procedure to Ning-kuo prefecture an alchemical adept." See footnote p. 154.

[9] Needham, J., Gwei-Djen, L. and Sivin, N. (2004). *Science and Civilisation in China, Vol 6-6 Biology and Biological Technology Medicine* (p. 134). United Kingdom: Cambridge University Press, 2004, 134.

[10] Timonius, E. and Woodward, J. (1753). *An Account, or History, of the Procuring the Small Pox by Incision, or Inoculation; As it Has for Some Time Been Practised at Constantinople, Philosophical Transactions* (Vol. 29., No. 339., p. 73). England: Royal Society of London

[11] Ibid.

[12] Prisoners on death row. They received an offer from the queen that whoever took part in the experiment would be pardoned. All six prisoners in the experiment willingly agreed to take part in it. They all survived and as promised, were released after experiment was over.

13 Johnson, Ben. (n.d.). *Newgate Prison Wall*. Retrieved from www.historic-uk.com/HistoryMagazine/DestinationsUK/Newgate-Prison-Wall/

[14] Behbehani, A.M. (1983). The Smallpox Story: Life and Death of an Old Disease. *Microbiological Reiews*, 47(4), 462.

[15] Creighton, C. (1894). *A History of Epidemics in Britain. Vol II From the Extinction of Plague to the present time* (p. 519). London: C.J. Clay, M.A and Sons, Cambridge University Press Warehouse.

CHAPTER 2

From magic to medicine

"Medicine is not only a science; it is also an art. It does not consist of compounding pills and plasters; it deals with the very processes of life, which must be understood before they may be guided."

~**Paracelcus** *(alchemist and physician).*

In Britain, The Royal Society of Medicine was interested in the various inoculation techniques used around the world. With a desire to educate themselves and put into practice efficient and safe inoculation methods, its members studied the methods used by other cultures. The society recorded their observations in an article:

> *"In India, before variolation, the subject to be inoculated had to undergo a strict dietetic régime and after the operation, which was performed upon the upper arm by placing wool dipped in smallpox secretion on a scratched surface, the patient had to live in the open, away from people, and on a light diet."*[1]

The Royal Society's members continued describing what they had learned about the methods the Chinese used and also the then-Siamese:

> *"In China, we are told, the inoculum consisted of smallpox crusts mixed with musk and rolled into a pledget of wool which was inserted into the nose, while in Siam the dried infective material was simply insufflated."*[2]

Insufflate, incidentally, means to breathe or blow vapor, air or a powdered medicine through or into a body cavity.

The genuine interest the scientific community of the day had in people's health is no better demonstrated than in the Royal Society of Medicine's obvious desire to discover the different inoculation methods already in use around the world. Its members pointed out that in India, the post dietary plan was used "to reduce the intensity of the smallpox reaction"[3]. This coincided with scientific data the society had which confirmed a correlation between diet and viral concentration.

As for the Chinese method, the guess was that the "musk containing essential oil"[4] was used to inhibit viral growth.

Russia, which had suffered greatly by the hands of smallpox, also seemed eager to learn from other cultures. In 1689, they sent students to China to learn about smallpox inoculation. Interestingly, though, when the Russian imperial family wanted to be inoculated, they did not turn to the Chinese. They asked Dr. Thomas Dimsdale, a Western doctor, to do it.[5]

As a further example of their keen interest in various methods the Royal Society of London published papers on the Chinese method in 1700, and in 1714 and 1716 on the Turkish method.[6]

Unfortunately, even though smallpox was rampaging, Britain's physicians held on to traditions and were slow to act on these alternative methods. The French were not on board with this inoculation process, either. They didn't practice it until it was pointed out to them that it could have saved them almost one million lives already.

Epidemics

Epidemics were frequent and people all over the world were frightened by them. In the 1545 smallpox epidemic in Goa, India, almost 8,000 children died. Entire villages were wiped out in the 1625 smallpox epidemic in North America. Another historical epidemic was the Massachusetts Colonial epidemic in 1633 where Governor William Bradford stated that an indian village by the Connecticut River with 1,000 inhabitants became devoured with the smallpox virus, in so much that 950 of them died.

In 1634, the governor of Massachusetts, John Wintrop, wrote to Sir Nathaniel Rich:

*"For the natives, they are neere all dead of the small Poxe,
so as the Lord hathe cleared our title to what we possess"[7].*

As tragic as this was, it was not considered a tragedy by all. One of those individuals was Reverend Increase Mather[8], who in 1632 saw the smallpox as a great blessing:

> *"About the same Time the Indians began to be quarrelsome touching the Bounds of the Land which they had sold to the English; but God ended the Controversy by sending the Small-pox amongst the Indians at Saugust, who were before that Time exceeding numerous. Whole Towns of them were swept away, in some of them not so much as one Soul escaping the Destruction."[9]*

Another smallpox plague in 1679 called the *Indian Plague*, took countless souls. In the words of Count de Frontenac Louis de Buade:

> *"The Small Pox desolates them to such a degree that they think no longer of Meeting nor of Wars, but only of bewailing the dead, of whom there is already an immense number."[10]*

The Western way

With smallpox ravaging the world, the desperation for a cure was understandable. By the early 18th Century, variolation was the most logical choice for prevention. It had become a common practice in the Western Hemisphere by 1721, but not without opposition.

Boston physician, Dr. Zabdiel Boylston, was a believer in the practice and performed experiments which in some instances ended in death. This caused uproar and people actively opposed the practice of variolation. Multiple pamphlets were written by both those for and against it.

In July, 1721, physicians and surgeons gathered together for a meeting. Together with His Majesty's Justices of the Peace and Select-Men, they decided against inoculation. Dr. Boylston was not pleased with their decision.

Their reasoning for taking a stand against inoculation, was as follows:

"IT appears by numerous Instances, That it has prov'd the Death of many Persons soon after the Operation, and brought Distempers upon many others which have in the End prov'd deadly to 'em.

"That the natural tendency of infusing such malignant Filth in the Mass of Blood, is to corrupt and putrify it, & if there be not a sufficient Discharge of that Malignity by the Place of Incision, or elsewhere, it lays a Foundation for many dangerous Diseases.

"That the Operation tends to spread and continue the Infection in a Place longer than it might otherwise be.

"That the continuing the Operation among us is likely to prove of most dangerous Consequence."[11]

The inoculation process was considered so dangerous that it wasn't legalized until after the aforementioned experiment on prisoners at Newgate in August 1721.

After this, when the inoculation process didn't go as planned, the *inoculators* would often push the blame away from themselves. Instead, they blamed the deaths on causes unrelated to the inoculation. This didn't sit well with those who opposed inoculations. Many doctors and clergy men ended up opposing the practice, and "[i]n 1722, an anonymous pamphlet appeared, which described inoculation as the outcome of atheism, quackery, and avarice."[12]

Dr. Wagstaffe, who worked as a doctor at St. Bartholomew's Hospital expressed his concerns regarding inoculations. These concerns are reminiscent of today's concerns regarding population control:

"Thus, the Operator has it in his power to convey the Small Pox to distant Places and Persons, who neither avow his practice or desire his experiment: And if 'tis possible that ingrafted Pox can be so poysonous as to communicate certain death to all around by this method, they may ingraft as violent a Plague as has been known among us. How far the Legislature may think fit to interpose, in order to prevent such an artificial way of depopulating a Country, is not my Province to determine. "[13]

The Boston inoculation party

Around the same time, a ship from the West Indies sailed into Boston harbor. Unbeknown to the passengers and Boston residents, she carried with her the smallpox virus. In Boston at this time, Reverend Cotton Mather (son of Rev. Increase Mather) was considered to have played an important role in the eradication of smallpox.

Rev. Mather had urged all of the physicians in the area to help inoculate the Bostonians. A physician answering his call was a Dr. Boylston. Together, they started inoculating the willing Bostoners.

The medical community in Boston was not pleased. It felt the inoculation would only spread the disease and not limit it. These inoculation-opposing physicians argued that Man shouldn't mingle in the Lord's affairs. This practice was so upsetting to the physicians, that they fought a legal battle against Dr. Boylston for "intentionally exposing citizens to a potentially fatal disease."[14] (Ironically, later on, many of these physicians published papers in favor of inoculation. The only thing that seemed to have changed, was that this time they had a financial gain in doing so).

A closer look at Rev. Mather reveals his earlier opinions were perhaps not far off from his medical opponents.' In fact, in his diary, we find passages about sins being the cause of illnesses:

> *"There are it may be Two Thousand Sicknesses: and indeed, any one of them able to crush us! But what is the Cause of all? Bear in Mind, That Sin was that which first brought Sickness upon a Sinful World, and which yett continues to sicken the World, with a World of Diseases."*[15]

Rev. Mather continues to preach about sickness being the result of the Original Sin when Adam and Eve ate the forbidden fruit. In other words, when we become sick, it is only a product of our sins.

He continues:

> *"Fools, because of their Transgression, and because of their Iniquities, are afflicted, with Sickness. Indeed Sin sometimes is Naturally the Cause of Sickness. A Sickness in the Spirit will naturally cause a Sickness in the Body."*[16]

When the news of smallpox outbreaks reached Rev. Mather, he saw it as a new disease brought upon us by God:

> *"It is one of those new Scourges whereof there are several, which the Holy and Righteous God has inflicted on a sinful World."*[17]

The authors of a study into Rev. Mather's diary entries, one of which is called *The Angel*, has a passage regarding childbirth. The authors share their interpretation of his words in dismay:

> *"Those in pain should remember that they are suffering for their sins, just as Christ suffered on the cross for the sins of all mankind. (In the chapter on childbirth, seventeen out of twenty-one pages are devoted to moralizing of this sort.) And the proper thoughts for smallpox victims are those of self-abhorrence and self-abasement: such creatures are to be viewed as loathsome."*[18]

Could Rev. Mather's change from persecuting the sick as sinners to saving people from sickness have something to do with the fact that, in 1713, three of Mather's children, his wife and maid were killed by measles[19]?

Chapter 2: From magic to medicine

[1] Ledingham, J.C.G. (1935). The Comparative Study of Clinically Allied Viruses: Some unsolved Problems of Edward Jenner. *Proceedings of the Royal Society of Medicine*, 29(2), 73-74.

[2] Ibid.

[3] Ibid.

[4] Ibid.

[5] Griffiths, J. (1984). Doctor Thomas Dimsdale, and Smallpox in Russia. *Bristol Medico-Chirurgical Journal*, January. Retrieved from www.europepmc.org/backend/ptpmcrender.fcgi?accid=PMC5077001&blobtype =pdf

[6] Fenner, F., Henderson, D.A., Arita., Jezek, Z., and Ladnyi, I.D. (1988). *Smallpox and its Eradication* (Table 6.1, p. 247). Geneva, Switzerland: World Health Organization.

[7] Winthrop, A., Winthrop, J.,Winthrop F. and Winthrop W. (1628). *Winthrop Papers* (p. 167). Boston: Massachusetts Historical Society.

[8] Harvard University. (n.d.). *Increase Mather*. Retrieved from www.harvard.edu/about-harvard/harvard-glance/history-presidency/increase-mather

[9] Mather, I. (1864). *Early History of New England* (pp. 110-111). Boston: Samuel G. Drake; and Albany, N.Y.: J. Munsell.

[10] The College of Physicians of Philadelphia. (n.d.). *The History of Vaccines*. Retrieved from www.historyofvaccines.org/content/indian-plague

[11] Boylston, Z. (1726). *An Historical Account of the Small-pox Inoculated in New England* (p. 53). London: Printed for S. CHANDLER, at the Cross-Keys in the *Poultry*. Edwards & Broughton.

[12] Crookshank, E. (1889). *History and Pathology of Vaccination, Vol I* (p. 39). London: H.K Lewis.

[13] Ibid. (p. 39-40).

[14] Gross, C.P. and Sepkowitz, K.A. (1998). The Myth of the Medical Breakthrough: Smallpox, Vaccination, and Jenner Reconsidered. *International Journal of Infectious Diseases*, 57.

[15] Beall, O., Shryock, R. (1968). *Cotton Mather: First Significant Figure in American Medicine* (p. 171). Baltimore: The John Hopkins Press.

[16] Ibid. (p. 172).

[17] Ibid. (p. 200).

[18] Ibid. (pp. 114-115).

[19] Hostetter, M.K. (2012). What We Don't See. *N Engl J Med*, 366, 1328-1334.

CHAPTER 3

The medicine man

*"To study the phenomena of disease without
books is to sail an uncharted sea, while to study
books without patients is not to go to sea at all."*

~*William Osler*.

In 1772, Englishman Edward Jenner had served as an apprentice to two surgeons for nine years. After his apprenticeships he "established himself as the local practitioner and surgeon."[1]

His credentials would be harshly criticized by his future opponents. One such opponent was the renowned Dr. Walter Hadwen. He may have been known for his anti-vaccine views, but he also had a degree in Surgery and Midwifery. He had also received multiple trophies such as:

> *"First Prizeman in Physiology, Operative Surgery,
> Pathology and Forensic Medicine, and also that of Suple
> Prizeman and double Gold Medallist in Surgery and
> Medicine."*[2]

In an 1896 address, during a smallpox epidemic in Gloucester, Dr. Hadwen demeaned Jenner's qualifications by saying:

> *"Jenner looked upon the whole thing as a superfluity, and
> he hung up 'Surgeon, apothecary,' over his door without
> any of the qualifications that warranted the assumption."*[3]

Dr. Hawden explained how Jenner received his degree of Doctor of Medicine from the Scotch University simply by paying them £15.

He then further attacks Jenner's character by stating that Dr. Norman Moore, who was Jenner's biographer, admitted that,

"[...] it was obtained by little less than a fraud. It was obtained by writing a most extraordinary paper about a fabulous cuckoo[4], for the most part composed of arrant absurdities and imaginative freaks such as no ornithologist of the present day would pay the slightest heed to."[5]

As if this wasn't enough, he continued on about Jenner's relentless attempts to acquire further degrees without any education:

"Jenner communicated with the University of Oxford and asked them to grant him their honorary degree of M.D., and after a good many fruitless attempts he got it. Then he sent to the Royal College of Physicians in London to get their diploma, [...]. [...] they considered he had quite enough on the cheap already, and told him distinctly that until he passed the usual examinations they were not going to give him any more."[6]

Edward Jenner never took any examinations and therefore never achieved a diploma as a physician.

Jenner is mostly recognized for his work on developing a smallpox vaccine. The story began in 1774 when rumors from rural people about cowpox preventing smallpox could be heard. This hypothesis had no scientific basis, it was merely a word of mouth storytelling. Jenner decided to test this theory by making a cut in the arm of a neighbor's eight-year-old son James Phipps. He then rubbed cowpox matter from a milkmaid's hand into it.

After two months, he made more incisions in both of James' arms and covered the cuts with smallpox pus from an infected person. The records say the boy did not contract smallpox. What we don't know, because it has never been noted in any reports, is whether the boy had previous exposure to smallpox.[7]

After 23 experiments, Jenner concluded that the cowpox matter gave humans immunity against the smallpox virus. He sent his discovery to the Royal Society, but they rejected his paper. He took it upon himself to publish the information in a brochure titled *An Inquiry into the Causes and Effects of the Variolae Vaccinae[8], a Disease discovered in some of the Western Counties of England, particularly Gloucestershire, and known by the name of Cow Pox.[9]*

This was the first time cowpox was referred to as *Variolae Vaccinae,* a term that Jenner conjured up. This new name was not mentioned anywhere else in the brochure.

Often when scholars or other medical professionals read scientific brochures, pamphlets or papers, they will only read the heading and the abstract. It's therefore not surprising that the phrase stuck. Many of them would have assumed this was the proper scientific name for cowpox.

In 1798, as Jenner continued his experimentations, he took samples from the sore of a stableman. He had become infected when cleaning grease[10] from the hooves of a horse. Jenner used a sample from the stableman's infection to inoculate the five-year-old John Baker.

Unfortunately, Jenner was not known for his detailed note-taking and only briefly described his observation of his experiment with John Baker, without any explanations, leaving the reviewers no knowledge of the experimental process. All he wrote was:

> *"He became ill on the 6th day with symptoms similar to those excited by Cow-Pox matter. On the 8th day he was free from indisposition [...] the boy was rendered unfit for inoculation from having felt the effects of a contagious fever in a work-house, soon after this experiment was made."*[11]

It appears suspicious that Jenner makes the conclusion, without explanation, that the boy's illness was due to the fever that was going around in the workhouse. The account is very poorly detailed, but from what Jenner states, six days after the inoculation, the boy became sick from something that looked like cowpox. Two days after that, he was no longer fit for inoculation (as we later find out, it was because the boy died). There is nothing that indicates the boy was already at the workhouse when inoculated, so we can only assume that he was sent to the workhouse after he fell sick and died there two days later. Especially when looking at the picture attached to his case. It has no date, but it tells a more serious story than Jenner's account, leaving experts in the field to believe the infection was more serious than he made it sound.

As we mentioned, Jenner didn't explain properly why the boy was unfit to continue the experiment until a year later, in the second edition of his pamphlet. This account can only be seen in a footnote. Misleadingly, this is found 60 pages past the actual case study. It doesn't mention the boy's name, merely refers to him as "Case xviii" and explains that:

"The boy unfortunately died of a fever at a parish workhouse before I had an opportunity of observing what effects would have been produced by the matter of Small Pox."[12]

Jenner's vaccine was eventually accepted. The risk of transferring disease was considered to be less likely with vaccination compared to variolation, which eventually tapered out and became illegal in Britain in 1840.

Edward Jenner received much opposition from people, including other doctors who felt his conclusion on cowpox building immunity towards smallpox was false. They had also seen people exposed to cowpox and afterwards become sick with smallpox all the same.

An example of this is the summary of a Gloucestershire Medical Society meeting in 1790. A society of which Jenner was one of the five founders:

"Baron says that at the meetings of this Society Jenner was wont to hold forth on the cow-pox question with such insistence that he was voted a bore by his fellow members, and finally threatened with expulsion if 'he continued to harass them with so unprofitable a subject.' Truly, there are some that having ears, yet hear not!"[13]

Such attacks must have frustrated Jenner quite a bit, because in 1798, he wrote in a letter to his friend, Mr. Edward Gardner:

"My friends must not desert me now. Brickbats and hostile weapons of every sort are flying thick around me; but with a very little aid, a few friendly opiates seasonably administered, they will do me no injury."[14]

Jenner didn't like his methods criticized. When smallpox broke out in Edinburgh 1818–19 and in Norwich in 1819, many of those who received Jenner's vaccine died. People started doubting the vaccine actually worked. Jenner's reaction was to steer the blame away from himself and the vaccines. Instead he pointed out that the vaccine must have been administered incorrectly.

Edgar Crookshank, an English physician and microbiologist[15] who favored the practice of variolation over vaccination, made a good point when he explained that even though variolation was "a dangerous practice," it was at least a scientific one because it entailed "the prevention or modification of a disease by artificially inducing a mild attack of that disease."[16]

But he said what Jenner was doing was artificially injecting people with a completely different disease, an idea that has never been scientifically supported.[17] At the end of his book, Crookshank makes a compelling statement:

> "Unfortunately, a belief in the efficacy of vaccination has been so enforced in the education of the medical practitioner, that it is hardly probable that the futility of the practice will be generally acknowledged in our generation [...] It is more probable that when, by means of notification and isolation, Small Pox is kept under control, vaccination will disappear from practice, and will retain only an historical interest."[18]

We find it very interesting that a man of his caliber and having been engrossed in the field of infectious diseases, would doubt vaccination efficacy so deeply as to make an official statement saying he does not believe the medical establishment would continue the practice in future.

Chapter 3: The medicine man

[1] The Jenner Institute. (n.d.). *About Edward Jenner.* Retrieved from www.jenner.ac.uk/edward-jenner

[2] Farnaud, S. (2009). The Dr Hadwen Trust for Humane Research: 39 years of Replacement Science. *ATLA,* 37(2), 39.

[3] Hadwen W. (1896). *The Case Against Vaccination.* [An address at Goddard's assembly rooms, Gloucester, Jan 25). Retrieved from www.soilandhealth.org/wp-content/uploads/02/0201hyglibcat/020119hadwin/020119hadwenrallytalk.html

[4] His "Cuckoo research" can be read in more detail in Dr. Charles Creighton's book: *Jenner and Vaccination: A Strange Chapter of Medical History.*

[5] Hadwen W. (1896). *The Case Against Vaccination.* [An address at Goddard's assembly rooms, Gloucester, Jan 25]. Retrieved from www.soilandhealth.org/wp-content/uploads/02/0201hyglibcat/020119hadwin/020119hadwenrallytalk.html

[6] Ibid.

[7] James Phipps is said to have died from consumption (Tuberculosis) at age 20. Jenner also vaccinated his son on more than one occasion, who also died of consumption at age 21. There have been arguments that link consumption to be an effect of the smallpox vaccine.

[8] Variolae Vaccinae means Smallpox of the cow. It is a misleading phrase used only in the heading. Not once does it appear in the pamphlet. Considering the fact that many scientists and physicians would only read the heading and the abstract, it erroneously, became widely assumed that cowpox was the same as smallpox of the cow.

[9] Jenner, E. (1798). *An Inquiry into the Causes and Effects of the Variolae Vaccinae.* [Pamphlet]. London: Sampson Low.

[10] Grease is an infection on the hooves of a horse.

[11] Jenner, E. (1798). *An Inquiry into the Causes and Effects of the Variolae Vaccinae.* [Pamphlet, p. 36]. London: Sampson Low.

[12] Jenner, E. (1802). *An Inquiry into the Causes and Effects of the Variolae Vaccinae.* [Pamphlet, p. 59]. Springfield: Ashley & Brewer.

[13] British Medical Association., Kirtland, G., McVail, John., John, C., Hime, T.W., and Royal College of Surgeons of England. (1896). Records of an old Medical Society: Some Unpublished Manuscripts of Edward Jenner. *The British Medical Journal,* 1298.

[14] Baron, J. (1838). *Life of Edward Jenner, M.D.* London: Henry Colburn,

[15] Wikipedia. (2018, June 6). *Edgar Crookshank.* Retrieved from www.en.wikipedia.org/wiki/Edgar_Crookshank

[16] Crookshank, E.M. (1889). *History and Pathology of Vaccination* (Vol. 1, p. 424). Philadelphia: P. Blackiston.

[17] Ibid (p. 464).

[18] Ibid (p. 465-466).

CHAPTER 4

Beginning of vaccine era

"We should not be afraid to go into a new era, to leave the old beyond."

~Zach Wamp (American politician).

Despite the *anti-vaccers'* efforts, the pro-vaccination campaign prevailed. European countries started traveling to other parts of the world with their new smallpox vaccine in hope of immunizing other cultures.

In this section we share with you an article we read in a paper[1] written on the historical account of a smallpox mission. This article shares the accounts from a journey sparked by an incident in 1798 when smallpox hit many members of the Spanish Bourbon royal family. King Charles IV reacted by making variolation a mandatory process in all of Spain.

Only two years after this announcement, the king heard that smallpox was ravaging the Spanish colonies. He prepared a warship stocked with the vaccine. There was only one problem: there was no way the vaccine would stay virulent during the trip since there were no refrigeration amenities or any other means to keep it sterile aboard ship.

This problem was solved by bringing along 22 orphaned children. Four nurses were hired to attend to them on board. These children had never had smallpox or been vaccinated for it.

The head nurse brought her own son to serve the same purpose as the orphans, which was to be human incubators.

The virus was transported in the children's fluid-filled blisters. When blisters started leaking fluid, the fluid would be passed on to the next child via skin contact. The fluid was then stored on "glass slides sealed with paraffin and subsequently stored using a vacuum technique that used pneumatic machines."[2]

At each port of call, they instituted a vaccination board and explained why it's important to vaccinate and set up local cowpox lymph production. They also vaccinated those willing and documented their work. They even designed an observation technique for any side-effects.[3]

Sounds like already back then, scientists were aware of issues with people reacting adversely to vaccines.

King Charles' smallpox vaccine champions were not popular in every port. When they reached Lima, Peru, they found vaccinations were already well established. The vaccination *business* paid local doctors quite well and they were not pleased to have newly-arrived visitors not charge for vaccinations.

The robbing of the lucrative mass vaccination business made the Spaniards unpopular among the Peruvian doctors. Fortunately for the Spaniards, it so happened Lima had just received a new viceroy who advocated on the Spaniards' behalf. They ended up vaccinating 197,000 people.

During their mission to vaccinate, the Spanish visitors encountered all kinds of problems—some political, others financial—and the resulting run-ins weren't always peaceful.

When the Spaniards arrived in Mexico, the opposition was so intense that a Mexican nurse advocating on behalf of vaccines was killed in the process.[4]

Meanwhile, back in the West

At this stage in history, all countries harbored the fear of diseases entering their cities. In 1799, Philadelphia's Board of Health built the Philadelphia Lazaretto Quarantine Station on Tinicum Island. Before entering Philadelphia, all travelers stricken with disease were quarantined at the station, which also served as a security/inspection station for all passengers and cargos headed for Philadelphia.[5]

The first person to vaccinate in the US was Benjamin Waterhouse who vaccinated his own children in 1800. He was a verbal advocate for vaccinations and wrote his previous university roommate, Founding

Father and President John Adams, to support him in informing people about the cowpox vaccine.

Waterhouse was concerned Adams wouldn't respond to him, so he sent Vice President Thomas Jefferson a pamphlet he had written called, *A prospect of exterminating the smallpox.* Jefferson replied on December 25, 1800 expressing great interest and praise. At one point he says, "Every friend of humanity must look with pleasure on this discovery [...]" and continues relating diseases to evil and vaccinations as helping get rid of evils.[6]

In 1802, Waterhouse tried to limit the distribution of vaccinations to himself, and only himself, so he could profit from other doctors by making the vaccine only available through him.

Instead of approaching Waterhouse for vaccines, the doctors found other ways to retrieve the ingredients. They would, for instance, collect pus from pustules of a vaccinated patient. This led to disaster when pus was collected from an unvaccinated British sailor and killed 68 people.

As the doctors kept finding their own sources, Waterhouse eventually started sharing his supply of vaccines.[7]

As mentioned, Thomas Jefferson was also a big vaccine advocate. After reading Jenner's paper, which he received from Rev. Dr. G.C. Jenner, Jefferson replied by thanking him on behalf of the "whole human family" and praised him in the highest regards for his discovery of something that "[m]edicine has never before produced any single improvement of such utility."[8]

The race

Since then, many scientists around the world started experimenting with vaccines for various illnesses. They were eager to find a way to improve the vaccine quality and prevent people from falling ill.

The race was on. Many competed to become the next big name in vaccine science.

For many scientists their names and reputations were at stake and the cost of losing detrimental. This didn't help in keeping them honest. Nor did it do anything to promote the reliability of their data.

To this day, after dozens of new vaccines have been introduced, pathogens, or microorganisms that can cause disease, still continue to spread and haunt us. Many of the struggles encountered in containing these germs are a by-product of our ever-evolving tighter living spaces. The more congested our cities and towns become, the easier it is for germs to survive. We spread these germs to those we come in contact with. This is *achieved* via a variety of means, including rapid population growth, trading and traveling, hygiene and sanitation or lack of, or depending on where you might live, wars, invasions and (modern-day) slavery. As our way of living evolves, our bodies strive to evolve with it.

Perhaps it is safe to assume that with better germ-growing conditions and with more toxins being introduced into the environment, our body will respond by adapting to these conditions. In the meantime, while our bodies are adapting, are the vaccines a good and safe way to stay healthy?

Chapter 4: Beginning of vaccine era
[1] Franco-Paredes, C., Lammoglia, L. and Santos-Preciado, J. (2005). The Spanish Royal Philanthropic Expedition to Bring Smallpox Vaccination to the New World and Asia in the 19th Century. *Clinical Infectious Diseases*, 41(9), 1285-1289. www.doi.org/10.1086/496930
[2] Ibid.
[3] Ibid.
[4] Ibid.
[5] The College of Physicians of Philadelphia. (n.d.). *The History of Vaccines*. Retrieved from www.historyofvaccines.org/no-view/philadelphia-lazaretto-built
[6] Waterhouse, B. (1802). *A Prospect of exterminating the Small Pox Part II* (p. 22). Cambridge: The University Press.
[7] The College of Physicians of Philadelphia. (n.d.). *The History of Vaccines* (Timeline: 1802 Vaccination Endorsed). Retrieved from www.historyofvaccines.org/timeline#EVT_60
[8] Buffalo, Public Library., Gluck, J.F., and Elmendorf, T.W. (1899). *Descriptive Catalogue of the Gluck Collection* (p. 64). Buffalo, New York: The Matthews-Northrup Co.

CHAPTER 5

Live/attenuated vaccines

"It's a pretty amazing to wake up every
morning, knowing that every decision I make is
to cause as little harm as possible. It's a pretty
fantastic way to live."

~*Colleen Patrick-Goudreau*

In a valiant attempt to protect us from harmful germs, scientists set out to invent new and improved vaccines. Some do it simply for the love of healing or scientific discovery, or both perhaps, while others are fired up by the pursuit of fame and recognition. We will leave their individual stories to other authors to cover, while we focus on scientists' acknowledged and patented childhood vaccines.

To cover as many of these (childhood vaccines) as possible, we have decided to use the vaccines on the US childhood schedule of the *Center for Disease Control and Prevention (CDC)*. This schedule, as far as we can tell, includes more vaccines than any other country in the world. If the vaccine is on the schedule, it will blanket other childhood vaccines used across the world. The main difference will be the manufacturer of the vaccines.

After looking at the various vaccines, we noticed they are not all the same. Some contain dead germs, some contain living germs while others have no germs at all. We figured there had to be a good reason for the different types of vaccines so we decided to make that a part of our research, thinking it would be an essential component in the bigger picture.

The vaccine types can be organized into four categories: live/attenuated (weakened) vaccines, inactivated/killed vaccines, toxoid vaccines and subunit/conjugate vaccines.[1]

Live/Attenuated vaccines

Some vaccines are manufactured by using the entire germ. Those are the live, attenuated vaccines. Attenuated because even though the virus is alive, it has been weakened in the lab so it won't replicate very well inside our body and make us sick.

Scientists are able to find a living germ to put into the vaccine by collecting it (the germ) from an individual infected by the wild version of it. A wild germ is a germ found out in nature. If it isn't wild, then it has been altered in the laboratory or is a descendant of a laboratory-altered germ.

Since it's a weakened form of the wild germ, it is considered to mimic the natural disease the most out of all the vaccines. This is also why it's considered to have the longest and the strongest immune response of them all.

The problem is, since it's a weakened, living germ, in order for it to work, it has to be able to replicate inside our body.[2] At the same time, we don't want it to replicate too fast because our immune system needs to be able to handle the attack.

Vaccine trials are done on healthy individuals. Let's say they measure the safe rate of replication for a healthy child and then use that same vaccine on a child with a compromised immune system. What appears to happen at times, is that some children have such a severely compromised immune systems that it causes the virus to replicate out of control.[3]

Vaccines that are manufactured this way are the rotavirus, measles-mumps-rubella (MMR), smallpox and chickenpox vaccines.

Technically, a virus is not a living thing, yet we consider them (viruses) living in terms of vaccines. Because virus is not alive, it can't replicate on its own. So, in order to produce live viral vaccines, living cells are needed in order to do the replication for it.

Bacteria, on the other hand, are living organisms. They don't need other living cells to grow as they can do that on their own. But what they do need are nutrients. Without proper nutrients or a suitable environment, they won't be able to multiply and, instead, they die.

Since viruses need living cells in order to replicate, when viral vaccines are made in the laboratory, they are grown in cultures which contain either human or animal cells.

Self-sufficient bacteria multiply and grow under the right conditions. In the laboratory, this means they are grown in cultures containing bacterial nutrition like sugar, protein or other important factors to control their pH level. The culture ingredients depend on the type of bacteria being grown.

As easy as this may sound, scientists sometimes have difficulty finding the perfect environment to culture and replicate their germs. There are some viruses that don't grow well on animal cells, but thrive on human cells. These are viruses that cause illnesses specific to humans, but don't infect other species when they are exposed. The smallpox virus would be an example of this.

Cell lines and cell strains

As mentioned, the viruses need living cells in order to replicate. Scientists often prefer human cells because the virus thrives better. Today, the two most commonly used human cell strains are WI-38 and MRC-5. By the way, cell strains and cell lines are two different things. Cell strains are produced using healthy cells while cell lines are produced using cancer cells.

WI-38 (Wistar Institute 38) are cells from the lung tissue of an aborted girl at three months gestation. It's used, for instance, in the manufacturing of MMR II, Varivax (chickenpox) and ProQuad (chicken pox & MMR).

MRC-5 cell strain (Medical Research Council cell strain 5) was developed in 1966 for the Medical Research Council (MRC) in England. This cell strain was cultured from lung tissue of an aborted baby boy at 14 weeks gestation. It is used in the manufacturing of such vaccines as Varivax (chicken pox), ProQuad (chicken pox & MMR), Havrix (Hep-A), Vaqta (Hep-A), DTaP, Hib and Polio (Pentacel).

These two strains, WI-38 and MRC-5, are human diploid cells. This means they have normal number of chromosomes and follow the *Hayflick[4] Limit[5]*. They can only replicate about 50 times before they die, as opposed to cancer cells which replicate endlessly.

An animal cell line used in vaccine making is the Vero cell line. Vero cells are kidney cells from the African green monkey and are grown in fetal bovine serum (FBS), which are cells from cows. This means that when the manufacturer uses Vero cells in making a vaccine, they are not only using monkey kidney cells, but also bovine cells. The rotavirus vaccine is grown in Vero cells. Vero is the splicing together of the words *Verda Reno,* which means *green kidney* in Esperanto (the international auxiliary language)[67].

Inside the blender

An example of how cells are used in vaccines is the polio vaccine from 1951. The book *Polio: an American story* describes the process using monkey kidneys. After the kidneys were removed:

> *"The cortex (outer layer) was then separated, chopped into tiny fragments, and 'rinsed several times with salt solution to remove blood and debris.'[...]"*[8]

After it had been chopped into tiny pieces, it was further isolated into single cells. They used a tissue culture called *Medium 199* which was made up of 60 different ingredients and was supposed to be the perfect nutrient for the monkey kidney cells. This may seem like a lot of ingredients, but the author asserts it was a better medium than what was used previously. He explains:

> *"Ever better, it did not contain the animal serums used in previous nutrient solutions, making it much safer for human use."* [9]

> *It sounds to us like he is saying it is better to use 60 ingredients than to grow the cells in fetal bovine serum.*

The live poliovirus was then inserted into the kidney cell culture medium. After a few days:

> *"[...] the mixture was harvested, placed in large glass bottles, and passed through a series of sensitive filters to screen out impurities. What emerged, in the end, were impressive quantities of pure, undiluted virus."*[10]

Now when the virus had been purified, it was time to pick the right strains. This was not an easy task:

> *"Some strains were potent but dangerous, others tired but safe. 'Essentially what is being searched for [...] is a (strain) powerful enough to cause immunity and yet docile enough to do no harm.'"*[11]

Jonas Salk explained the process of choosing strains:

> *"'We just put them in a race [...] Three of them gave brilliant, startling results, destroying monkey and human tissue right before our eyes. It was thrilling.'"*[12]

Salk was so sure of his ways that he picked the most destructive strains. These strains were then inactivated by using formaldehyde (FA). In order to test the strains to see if they had used too much or too little formaldehyde, they injected the monkeys with the formaldehyde-treated virus:

> *"[...] and watched for signs of polio. If even one took sick, the entire batch was destroyed. If all went well, the monkeys were sacrificed a month later and microscopically examined for any invasion of poliovirus."*[13]

Vaccines may not be made exactly like this today, but the idea regarding how to use the cells in a culture follows similar logic.

Uninvited guests

Many people think it's unethical to use human fetal cells in vaccine manufacturing. But there's a problem with using animal cells as well. Animals carry a wide selection of viruses that are foreign to we humans. We may not even know of all viruses that exist.

Mark Lipsitch[14], a Harvard Professor of Epidemiology said:

> *"'we can't predict what a virus we've never seen will do.'"*[15]

Since we're not really aware these viruses exist, we don't know how they will affect the human body when injected, nor do we know how to test for them. These unintended viruses are often called *passenger viruses*.

The Rubella strain (RA 27/3) used in the MMR vaccines is grown in WI-38. If you look it up on the Internet, there are countless articles expressing outrage over using these aborted human fetal cells to make the rubella vaccine.

The dilemma is that a virus has to be grown in living cells. We also learned animal cells carry viruses that can cause damage to our health. In order to make a vaccine as safe as possible for us, the scientists opted for human cells.

Dr. Stanley A. Plotkin[16], a renowned scientist, known for, among other things, the development of the rubella vaccine,[17] wrote in one of his papers:

> *"In order to avoid the problem of passenger viruses, the RA 27/3 strain was isolated directly from naturally infected material in WI-38 human diploid fibroblasts."*[18]

The concern scientists had regarding passenger viruses was not unfounded. You may recall the disastrous SV40 monkey virus which contaminated the polio vaccines. There are scientists who claim this virus is the cause of multiple human cancers.

On CDC's website a page on *vaccine safety*, which was suddenly removed (archived copies exist), states that:

> *"SV40 virus has been found in certain types of cancer in humans, but it has not been determined that SV40 causes these cancers."*[19]

Multiply and replenish

The live virus goes through a couple of hundred cycles or replications when in human or animal cell cultures. For each cycle, the virus weakens slightly. The goal is to get the virus strong enough to cause immunity, but too weak to cause disease. So, the number of cycles may differ for each vaccine. After the virus has gone through all these cycles, and changed a little bit each time, it has changed or evolved enough to adjust to its new environment in the laboratory. The virus is no longer a wild strain, but rather a vaccine strain.

During this long evolutionary process, the virus is not exposed to the human body and is therefore not considered to be of any harm to us. Not only will it no longer cause disease, but it replicates very poorly in our body. This makes it easier for our immune system to be in control.

When dealing with a living germ, we should also be aware that it can mutate. This is known to happen with live virus vaccines. The viruses have the ability to revert back to being harmful to us. It's difficult to know what the virus is capable of when it finds the opportunity to replicate within our body. This isn't supposed to happen, because the virus is very poor at replicating at this point. The problem arises when the virus actually does wake up, and history tells us it can happen.

Chapter 5: Live/attenuated vaccines

[1] U.S. Food and Drug Administration. (2018, May 9). *Vaccines for Children - A Guide for Parents and Caregivers*. Retrieved from www.fda.gov/BiologicsBloodVaccines/ucm345587.htm

[2] Center for Disease Control and Prevention. (n.d.). *Immunology and Vaccine-Preventable Diseases*. Retrieved from www.cdc.gov/vaccines/pubs/pinkbook/downloads/prinvac.pdf

[3] Center for Disease Control and Prevention. (n.d.). *General Recommendations on Immunization*. Retrieved from www.cdc.gov/vaccines/pubs/pinkbook/downloads/genrec.pdf

[4] The Embryo Project Encyclopedia. (2014, July 20). *Leonard Hayflick (1928-)*. Retrieved from www.embryo.asu.edu/pages/leonard-hayflick-1928

[5] The Embryo Project Encyclopedia. (2014, November 12). *The Hayflick Limit*. Retrieved from www.embryo.asu.edu/pages/hayflick-limit

[6] World Association For Vaccine Education (WAVE). (n.d.). *African Green Monkey Kidney Cells*. Retrieved from www.novaccine.com/vaccine-ingredients/african-green-monkey-kidney-cells/

[7] Wikipedia. (2018, December 15). *Esperanto*. Retrieved from www.en.wikipedia.org/wiki/Esperanto

[8] Oshinsky, D. (2006). *Polio: An American Story* (p. 154). United Kingdom: Oxford University Press.

[9] Ibid.

[10] Ibid. (p. 155).

[11] Ibid.

[12] Ibid.

[13] Ibid. (p. 156).

[14] Harvard T.H. Chan. (n.d.). *Faculty and Research Directory*. Retrieved from www.hsph.harvard.edu/marc-lipsitch/

[15] James, S. M. (2005, September 30). *How Many People Could Bird Flu Kill?*. Retrieved from www.abcnews.go.com/Health/Flu/story?id=1173856

[16] National Foundation for Infectious Diseases (NFID). (n.d.). *Stanley A. Plotkin, MD*. [Award]. Retrieved from www.nfid.org/awards/plotkin.pdf

[17] Buckley, M. (2009, July 01). *MTS30 - Stanley Plotkin - The Past, Present, and Future of Vaccines*. Retrieved from www.asm.org/index.php/podcasts/meet-the-microbiologist/item/3002-mts30-stanley-plotkin-the-past-present-and-future-of-vaccines

[18] Plotkin, S.A., Farquhar, J.D., Katz, M. and Buser, F. (1969). Attenuation of RA 27/3 Rubella Virus in WI-38 Human Diploid Cells. *Amer J Dis Child*, 118

[19] Centers for Disease Control and Prevention. (2007, October 22). *Vaccine Safety*. Retrieved from www.web.archive.org/web/20130522091608/http://www.cdc.gov/vaccinesafety/updates/archive/polio_and_cancer_factsheet.htm or www.cdc.gov/vaccinesafety/updates/archive/polio_and_cancer_factsheet.htm (This page has been removed).

CHAPTER 6

Altered germs

"Without laboratories men of science are soldiers without arms."

~Louis Pasteur *(French biologist)*

Some inactivated vaccines use the entire germ, while others use disease-causing portions of the germ. In vaccines containing the whole germ, scientists will inactivate or kill the germ in order to prevent viral replication. They do this by using chemicals. A chemical that's very good at this job is formaldehyde (FA) or formalin (liquid form of FA).

Even though the germ is killed and can no longer replicate, it's still whole, so our immune system is able to recognize it and attack it.

Unfortunately, the killed germ doesn't keep our body immune as long as a living germ will, so we need to get booster shots every so often to keep the immune response up. Examples of vaccines using killed germs are Hepatitis A and polio (shot).

Inactivated toxins (toxoids) vaccine

When the disease is caused by bacteria, it's often not the actual bacteria itself causing the sickness, but rather a toxic component of the bacteria. The goal of this vaccine is to inactivate the toxic component (toxoid), so it can be injected into our body without harming it. Toxoids are not quite the same as toxins. Toxins are the pure product of the bacteria and toxoids are the toxins after they have been chemically altered or inactivated in the lab. Examples of toxoid vaccines are diphtheria and tetanus.

Subunit/conjugate/recombinant vaccine

The differences between these types of vaccines (subunit/conjugate/recombinant) doesn't seem to be clearly understood by many we've come across in the medical field.

Subunit vaccines use only portions of the germ or as the NIH website explains it, they "include only the antigens that best stimulate the immune system."[1]

The conjugate vaccines, on the other hand, use only the bacterial sugar coat in order to "disguise a bacterium's antigens so that the immature immune systems of infants and younger children can't recognize or respond to them."[2] The coating also contains the information that makes us sick.

But this is not an actual germ, so if it is just injected into the body by itself, we won't recognize how dangerous the coating is. To solve this problem, the scientists attach it to a toxic molecule that will stir up our immune system. In order to attach the coating to the toxin, they need other chemicals to finish the job. By using a chemical, the coating material attaches to a carrier protein. Examples of these types of vaccines are the Hib, HPV, pneumococcal and meningococcal vaccines.

The recombinant vaccines, use carriers or vectors "to introduce microbial DNA to cells of the body."[3] These carriers/vectors are weakened viruses or bacteria, meaning they mix and match DNA from different sources into one germ or cell.

There are different ways to produce these vaccines. One way is to isolate a specific piece from a germ and use it in the vaccine. Another way is via genetic engineering. Here the germ is inserted into plasmid that has been manipulated by scientists. This type of plasmid is circular segments of DNA extracted from bacteria to serve as a vector. Scientists can add multiple genes and whatever genes they want into this plasmid. In case of vaccines, this includes a genetic piece of the vaccine germ and normally a gene for antibiotic resistance.

This means that when the toxic gene is cultured inside the yeast, it has been designed with a new genetic code that makes it resistant to the antibiotic it's coded for.

The gene-plasmid combo is inserted into a yeast cell to be replicated. When the yeast replicates, the DNA from the plasmid is reproduced as a part of the yeast DNA. Once enough cells have been replicated, the genetic material in the *new and improved* yeast cell is extracted and put into the vaccine. Examples of this vaccine are the acellular pertussis and hepatitis B vaccines.

One thing that doesn't seem to concern scientists is the fact that the manmade genetic combination becomes the vaccine component. This mixture of intended and unintended genetic information may cause our immune system to overreact. This can be especially complicated for a child with compromised immune system.

Another concern is that this new genetic code can become integrated with our own genetic material. Yeast, for instance, is very much like human DNA. It shares about one third of our proteins.

What have they done?

Here you have substances that are designed to aggravate the immune system towards an attack. So, that's what it does. Our immune system launches an attack on the invader. Sometimes the invader, like yeast, has many of the same protein codes as us. Our immune system downloads these protein codes and labels them as enemies. It signals a full-on attack on everything with that code in our body. Unfortunately, when the codes are similar, we don't always know how to distinguish between vaccine proteins and our own proteins.

Trace elements

Trace components that end up in the final product and become a part of the vaccine are usually left-over elements from the manufacturing process. These components were added during production in order to either keep cells alive or kill them or keep them free from contamination or to alter genetic materials during production. Other components are added to stir up our immune system to respond to the vaccine. As you perhaps can see, the materials scientists purposely add to the vaccine-making process serve the purpose of keeping us as safe as possible.

The concern arises when these materials become a danger to our body, which becomes overwhelmed from being bombarded with toxins and protein particles. This attack is, for some children, too much to handle, and they suffer permanent ill health or lose the fight to live.

What is it exactly that ends up in the vaccines our children are given, and what happens when these vaccines enter their bodies? We attempt to answer these questions in the next chapter.

Chapter 6: Altered germs

[1] World Health Organization. (n.d.) *Module 2: Types of Vaccine and Adverse Reactions.* Retrieved from www.vaccine-safety-training.org/subunit-vaccines.html

[2] Ibid.

[3] Ibid.

CHAPTER 7

Our own army of superheroes

"Birds born in cages think that flying is a disease."

~Alejandro Jodorowsky (Chilean-French filmmaker)

The vaccines entering the body come fully loaded with *heavy artillery*. Not all vaccine ingredients are well behaved, but rather are prone to vandalism once inside the body. In their defense, these ingredients are put in the vaccines because of their ability to ravage.

Whether the scientists intended it to or not, the vaccines are quite effective in causing the body to react in a way nature did not prepare it for. Most of the vaccine ingredients and trace elements are added in order to provide safety and efficacy. Each vaccine is different and comes with its own recipe and ingredients. So far, regardless of which vaccine it is or which recipe is used, our immune system reacts accordingly.

The body is extremely methodological in its defense/attack strategies. As authors, we felt it was very important to understand how some of these strategies work. The immune system is an extremely intelligent and intricate mechanism and we cannot possibly do it justice in only a few pages. In this chapter we share a fraction of its intricate puzzle, but hopefully it's enough to make sense of how our bodies are designed to react when presented with foreign substances.

Concepts such as the immune system adjusting to a growing fetus bring to mind other instances that may have had similar outcomes. The body adjusts to the germs in the environment and is able to protect itself from these germs and even draw benefits from them.

Sometimes the germs are so clever at surviving and upholding their genetic makeup they become a part of our human DNA.

A recent article at Livescience.com[1] mentions some research papers on how ancient viruses could be the reason humans have conscious thoughts, a functioning immune system and are able to develop embryo.

Another interesting finding the article points out is that we have a viral gene called the Arc gene[2]. This gene plays an important role in writing genetic information and getting it across to other neurons. It's so important, in fact, that without it, synapses will fade away. (A synapse is the area where the nerve signalling takes place: From the axon terminal, across the synaptic cleft and over to the dendrite). People who have been diagnosed with autism or other atypical neural diseases have been shown to have a dysfunctioning Arc gene.

Having read some of the massive amount of information on vaccines and related topics, we do wonder if our bodies would have evolved in such a way to withstand the diseases that concern us today *without* help of drugs or vaccines.

We understand that even before vaccinations, diseases killed huge numbers of people all over the world. As we mentioned at the end of the first chapter, when populations grew and people started living closer together, germs had more opportunities to spread amongst humans, especially where sanitation was a major problem. So, it makes us wonder if with improved living conditions would these diseases have been such a big issue? Did scientists become too focused on being a part of the medical revolution to see that perhaps the real solution lies in improving our environment?

The story of surgeon Ignas Semmelweis, who claimed washing hands would make childbirth much safer, is one example of improving the environment. He is now known for the *recognize-explain-act* approach, which is still used today as an epidemiological model for preventing infections.[3]

Chapter 7: Our own army of superheroes
[1] Letzter, R. (2018, February 2). *An Ancient Virus May Be Responsible for Human Consciousness.* Retrieved from www.livescience.com/61627-ancient-virus-brain.html
[2] www.genecards.org/cgi-bin/carddisp.pl?gene=ARC
[3] WHO Guidelines on Hand Hygiene in Health Care: First Global Patient Safety Challenge Clean Care Is Safer Care. Geneva: World Health Organization; 2009. 4, Historical perspective on hand hygiene in health care. Available from: www.ncbi.nlm.nih.gov/books/NBK144018/

CHAPTER 8

The helper cell

"The best advisers, helpers and friends,
always are not those who tell us how to act in
special cases, but who give us, out of themselves,
the ardent spirit and desire to act right, and
leave us then, even through many blunders, to
find out what our own form of right action is."

~Phillips Brooks (American clergyman and
preacher).

When a woman is pregnant, she carries a fetus which has its own sets of cells, its own DNA. It is its own individual being, which presents a problem for the immune system as it is designed to attack whatever is foreign in the body. This is an issue humans have dealt with since the beginning of time.

Nature has forced the female body to adapt and accept new life growing within. The body has had a long time to evolve and improve. Long enough that it now has the mechanisms in place to deal with the conundrum of new life smoothly. Nature itself has prepared the female body to allow a foreign entity to grow inside it.

In order to protect itself, the body uses many types of immune cells. One type is something called T-helper (Th or helper) cells. We have many different kinds of helper cells and their functions are distinguished by adding numbers to their names.

The most significant Th cells in relation to this book are the Th1 and Th2 cells. The main function of a Th1 cell is to help destroy our cells already infected by germs. The Th2 cells balance this out by helping destroy the germs outside the cells before they get the chance to attack them. This creates a Th1/Th2 cell balance. In other words, Th1 cells recognize your infected cells and help kill them before they produce other corrupted cells. The Th2 cells recognize the free-floating germs and help create antibodies against them.

In the case of the fetus, the Th1 cells are the problem. These cells believe the fetal cells are corrupt, so they signal an attack to destroy them. Since life has continued on this planet for who knows how long, it's apparent that nature has taught the body to bypass this fetal destruction. The body's immune system restructures its purpose in order to protect the fetus. It does this by suppressing the production of Th1 cells until after birth[1]. This way, the body doesn't have enough Th1 cells to attack what it believes to be corrupted cells.

This means the Th1/Th2 balance is interrupted and the future mother now has tipped the scales towards Th2 cells. This also means the mother has mostly Th2 cells and very little Th1 cells available to share with the fetus. Therefore, the placenta transfers almost entirely Th2 cells to the fetus.

It should come as no surprise that when we are born our immune system consists almost completely of Th2 cells. It's not until the baby is exposed to the outside environment that Th1 cells become stimulated and start multiplying until they become a balanced part of the immune system again.

We rely almost entirely on our mother's antibodies until we are about six months old, which is when we slowly start developing a more complex immune system. As a baby starts building its own immunity, the mother's antibodies disappear from the baby's body.

Something we weren't quite able to figure out was why babies receive so many vaccines before they start creating their own antibodies. A vaccine is meant to encourage the body to create antibodies against it. We can see how vaccinating an infant that's not good at creating its own antibodies yet, would only have limited protective effects. We also wondered whether the vaccine would therefore have a different effect on the infant than it would on a child with a fully developed immune system. Although we came up short on some of these concerns, we were able to get some answers we'll share with you in this book.

Hunt, eat and destroy

The first line of defense is the surface of our skin. The average skin pH is 4.7, which is acidic and ideal for our normal skin flora[2]. Another acidic location is our gut. Those of you who are gardeners will likely know how difficult it can be to grow plants in an acidic environment. It's the same with germs. Many germs don't survive being in contact with such acidic environment.

If the skin is compromised in any way, an open cut for instance, it will allow germs to make their way inside. This is where the germs meet our macrophages (i.e. phagocytes). They are called phagocytes because they eat everything foreign (phago = eat, cyte = cell). They are the first ones to the scene and will grab hold of the invaders then devour and destroy them. They don't distinguish between the foreign particles. They don't care what it is, as long as it's foreign. The macrophages then gather genetic information about the invader and bring it to the lymph nodes where the T cells and B cells hang out.

A quick recap: The T cells in question are the Th1 and Th2 cells. Th1 cells help destroy the infected cells and the Th2 cells help B cells make antibodies to inactivate the germs floating around outside our cells.

We never forget

As we just mentioned, B cells and Th2 cells work together in antibody production.

Some B cells go by the name of *memory cells* because they remember information about the invader for the rest of our lives (or close thereto). This means that when the same invader attacks again, the memory B cells are alerted much quicker. The B cells carrying the information begin cloning themselves and start spitting out antibodies at a much faster rate.

It will not pass

In nature, a germ is introduced to the body via the mucosal route such as the eye, nose or throat. When antigens (foreign invaders) enter the body naturally, the first defenders, which are a part of the innate immune system, respond instantaneously.

Vaccines are designed to skip the first responders (innate immunity) and go straight for the antibody producing responders (acquired immunity).

What's worth noting is if a vaccine manufacturer states that its vaccine elicits T cell response, it doesn't necessarily mean the vaccine elicits response from all types of T cells. This is because there are different types of T cells.

We have explained that Th1 and Th2 are *promoting* an action and not actually performing the task itself. Hence the name *helper cell*. Like the Th1 cells. When we look at their function a little closer, their job is to relay instructions that tell *Killer-T cells* what to do. The Killer-T cells receive the instructions, multiply themselves until they are an army carrying the same instructions and then they go kill the corrupted cells they were instructed to kill.

Once the Killer-T cells have destroyed corrupted cells, the macrophages come over to clean up the mess. The same goes for the Th2 cells. They carry instructions for the B-cells. After receiving instructions, the B cells will multiply until they are an army of cells carrying the same instructions.

What good is a titer?

The way physicians check to make sure your body has become properly immunized against a specific disease is to send you to the lab for a blood draw. Then your blood will be tested for the presence of the antibodies against specific antigens. A quick reminder, B cells produce antibodies.

When checking for vaccine immunity, the antibodies are often measured in *titers*. When we learned how vaccine immunity is measured in titers, we knew it was measuring the activity of Th2 cells and the B cells. What was completely missing was the activity performed by the Th1 cells and the Killer-T cells.

Given the way vaccinations are presented to our system, it seems to us there may be other factors than antibody concentration to consider. We found an interesting older study in *The Lancet* that tested individuals who were unable to produce their own antibodies[3]. When these individuals came down with measles, they showed all the natural signs and symptoms of natural disease. After the course of the illness, they became immune to measles.

The scientists conducting this study had blood drawn from these patients and tested it for antibody levels. There were no antibodies for measles in the blood (serum) samples. This goes to show that the immune system can create immunity against a disease without producing antibodies. And this means the immunity had nothing to do with Th2 cells or B cells, which are a part of the acquired (adaptive) immunity.

This study could be an example of the great importance of our first responders, the innate immune response, which reacts to the initial exposure of a disease. Our innate immune system is nonspecific, it attacks anything foreign. Our acquired immunity, the one that produces antibodies, the one lacking in the individuals in above study, consists of cells which only attack what they're instructed to attack.

The adjuvant rejuvenant

Most vaccines contain either inactivated germs or portions germs—an antigen nonetheless. If it were to be injected into the body all by itself, nothing would happen. It would just float uselessly around and the body wouldn't view it a threat.

The immune system needs to be artificially triggered and tricked into attacking these useless invaders. As a solution to this problem, scientists came up with the idea of attaching a substance to the vaccine antigen that would trigger B cells to produce antibodies. This substance is called an adjuvant.

Up until the early 2000s, mercury was often used as an adjuvant. As a result of some severe consequences and pressure from concerned citizens, mercury was eliminated from most vaccines.

The scientists knew the vaccine still needed an adjuvant if it was going to elicit an immune response. So, they added aluminum (Al) instead to do the job.

An adjuvant is designed to shock the B cells (and Th2 cells) into antibody production. Each vaccine antigen is coated with an adjuvant.

This raised two important questions for us: How many antigens are there in a vaccine; and when injecting multiple vaccines simultaneously, could this accumulation of adjuvants be more harmful—especially for infants?

Unfortunately, there are far too many antigens in a vaccine to be counted.

When adjuvants trigger antibody production for multiple antigens, the B cells are instructed to produce a wide variety and magnitude of antibodies. Keep in mind, it isn't natural for the body to be exposed to a variety of diseases all at the same time, especially all bypassing the innate immune system (first responders). And yet how many times have you heard of children being naturally sick with multiple childhood diseases all at the same time?

The CDC's recommended childhood vaccine schedule[45] recommends 69 shots up until age 18. This is *not* 69 different diseases. As you may recall, some vaccines require booster shots, so this count includes each booster as well. Some of these will be combined in the same vaccine. For example, measles, mumps & rubella (MMR) would be considered three shots as would diphtheria, tetanus & acellular pertussis (DTaP).

If the foreign antigens are too numerous and overpower the immune system, they will have the opportunity to run wild, and multiply within the body and vandalize it. Whatever the body is unable to eliminate stays there.

Once the vaccine ingredients are inside the body, is the body able to take care of them? Are they being excreted or are they accumulating? If they are accumulating, where are they, where are they going and are they causing damage? We hope to satisfactorily answer these questions and more in the coming chapters.

Chapter 8: The helper cell

[1] Sykes, L., MacIntyre, D. A., Yap, X. J., Ponnampalam, S., Teoh, T. G., & Bennett, P. R. (2012). Changes in the Th1:Th2 cytokine bias in pregnancy and the effects of the anti-inflammatory cyclopentenone prostaglandin 15-deoxy-Δ(12,14)-prostaglandin J2. *Mediators of inflammation*, 2012, 416739.

[2] Lambers H., Piessens, S., Bloem, A., Pronk, H., and Finkel, P. (2006). Natural skin surface pH is on average below 5, which is beneficial for its resident flora." *International Journal of Cosmetic Science*, 28(5), 359-370.

[3] Burnet F.M. (1968). Measles as an Index of Immunological Function. *The Lancet*, 292(7568), 610-613.

[4] Centers for Disease Control and Prevention. (2018, May 14). *Recommended Immunization Schedule for Children and Adolescents Aged 18 Years or Younger, United States, 2018*. Retrieved from www.cdc.gov/vaccines/schedules/hcp/child-adolescent.html

[5] Center for Disease Control. (n.d.). *Recommended Immunization Schedule for Children and Adolescents Aged 18 Years or Younger, UNITED STATES, 2018*. Retrieved from www.cdc.gov/vaccines/schedules/downloads/child/0-18yrs-child-combined-schedule.pdf

CHAPTER 9

Aluminum, it's getting on my cells

*"...Designers are generally unaware of the
effects that their inventions have on the brain,
and therefore take no responsibility of this role is
deeply worrying. The world of design is like a
highway, where each and every driver is asleep
at the wheel."*

~ *Jan Golembiewski (From the novel*
Magic)

Each manufacturer (of vaccines) has his or her own recipe for a particular
vaccine. But certain ingredients appear to be as popular as flour is to
baking. One of those popular, across-the-board-ingredients, as long as it
is not a live/attenuated vaccine, is the aluminum (Al) adjuvant.

Aluminum is a neurotoxin and the most commonly used adjuvant
today. It comes in the form of salts or gels. It irritates our immune system,
causing it to attack the invading germ or antigen it's attached to.

We have phosphate on our DNA. Aluminum attaches itself to it and
messes up our genetic coding process. While the aluminum is inside a cell,
some of its particles attach to adenosine triphosphate (ATP). The ATP is
in charge of our cell's energy production. So, in this manner the aluminum
can affect our energy level.

We have enzymes (proteins) within our cells that depend on attaching
themselves to calcium (Ca) or magnesium (Mg) to function properly.
Once our enzymes have attached to the Ca and Mg, they can carry on
with their functions.

Because the aluminum has such a strong positive charge, it's able to break the bond between our enzymes and Ca or Mg. These enzymes are now no longer attached to Ca or Mg. They have become neutralized and are unable to carry out their responsibilities. We need these enzymes for efficient metabolism, but now the aluminum is attached to the enzymes instead.

The protein molecules all look a little different because their shape reflects what they are designed to do. Aluminum disturbs their individual tasks and clumps them together so they are now misshapen and no longer functioning.

Aluminum also messes with the cell surface (the membrane) which is the outer layer of the cell. With a dysfunctional cell membrane, everything inside the cell becomes compromised and it is no longer able to properly communicate with the environment surrounding the cell about what needs to be done.[1]

It's all up in my brain

According to our research, one of the most knowledgeable scientists on the element aluminum would be Professor Chris Exley[2]. According to his profile on Keele University's website, since 1984 his research has been focused on the question "'how come the third most abundant element of the Earth's crust (aluminium) is non-essential and largely inimcal to life.'"[3]

Professor Exley has written multiple book-chapters and articles on aluminum and silicon. He has listed 98 published articles in peer-reviewed journals[4] on this subject. In November 2017, he wrote a blog post in *The Hippocratic Post*, which is "[t]he world's first global blogging site specializing in medical issues"[5], headed *Aluminum and autism*[6].

In that article he mentions a paper later published in 2018:

> *"The aluminum content of brain tissue in autism was consistently high. [...]*
>
> *These are some of the highest values for aluminium in human brain tissue yet recorded."*[7]

Inflammation is a big part of how our immune cells respond to attacks by foreign invaders. You may also recall how phagocytes clean up and help eliminate invaders. A type of phagocyte in the body is the monocyte.

Regarding aluminum, monocytes, autism spectrum disorder (ASD) and vaccines, Professor Exley concludes in his blog post:

> *"Perhaps there is something within the genetic make-up of specific individuals which predisposes them to accumulate and retain aluminium in their brain, as is similarly suggested for individuals with familial Alzheimer's disease. The new evidence strongly suggests that aluminium is entering the brain in ASD via pro-inflammatory cells which have become loaded up with aluminium in the blood and/or lymph, much as has been demonstrated for monocytes at injection sites for vaccines including aluminium adjuvants. Perhaps we now have the putative link between vaccination and ASD, the link being the inclusion of an aluminium adjuvant in the vaccine."* [8]

The attack on aluminum

We have established that aluminum can destroy the surface of a cell. The cell's components can now leak out. Once they are out of the cell, some of our immune cells, such as the phagocytes, will come to the scene and pick up the aluminum together with other debris that leaked out of the cells. As they gobble everything up, the phagocytes become filled with aluminum.

Using the information brought to them by the phagocytes, the T cells will delegate work to other members of the immune system. Some of those cells are called Th17 cells. These are cells responsible for inducing inflammation and bringing macrophages to the site. Remember, these macrophages may already have ingested aluminum.

Aluminum (Al) really aggravates this immune process, which is why it's used as an adjuvant in vaccines. The aluminum continues agitating the immune process repeatedly until it overloads our system. With the Th17 cells causing inflammation and the aluminum being where the inflammation is, it (the Al) just keeps triggering the Th17 cells to flare up the inflammation.[9]

Some of the material inside the cell is acidic and inflammatory. This is a great defense mechanism within the cell against pathogens. It's not so great when the cells leak, adding to the constant inflammation that's occurring. When this happens, our immune system is back on duty working hard to clean up the fragmented spill, which includes more aluminum.

Purely toxic

It's very important the person being vaccinated has healthy kidneys as they are a vital part of eliminating aluminum (Al) from the blood.

We wonder if many doctors test infants and children for healthy kidneys before vaccinating them. A good test for this would be to check the Glomerular Filtration Rate (GFR)[10]. This tells us how well the kidneys (glomerulus) are filtering the blood. To know how much aluminum the kidneys can handle, we must know their GFR.

One of the research papers we found on aluminum states in the first paragraph:

> *"[...] Al is invariably toxic to living systems and has no known beneficial role in any biological systems."* [11]

Later in the same paragraph it continues to warn:

> *"It injures cells, circuits, and subsystems and can cause catastrophic failures ending in death. Al forms toxic complexes with other element, such as fluorine, and interacts negatively with mercury, lead, and glyphosate. Al negatively impacts the central nervous system in all species that have been studied, including humans."*[12]

Aluminum placebo

The same research paper also mentions that in vaccine trials, the placebo for the control group is often an aluminum-containing vaccine. That fact alone could account for why so many mainstream-approved research studies have inconclusive and perhaps even contradictory outcomes.

How can you study the effect of a vaccine when its placebo (control) is an aluminum-based vaccine and not a pure saline solution as a true placebo is supposed to be? The paper uses an analogy to explain that using aluminum (Al) in a control group is like "comparing fire A against fire B, to make the argument that since A is no hotter than B, A is therefore not a fire."[13]

A 2011 paper, published in *PubMed*, by two of the authors of the above-mentioned paper, also states concerns about aluminum being used as an adjuvant in vaccines:

> *"Experimental research, however, clearly shows that aluminum adjuvants have a potential to induce serious immunological disorders in humans. In particular, aluminum in adjuvant form carries a risk for autoimmunity, long-term brain inflammation and associated neurological complications [...]."*[14]

We noticed when researching narrow subjects, it's often the same authors involved in much of the research. This is unfortunate, as it would be great to have reliable data from various authors.

Another study on aluminum, by the same authors as above, from 2013 states:

> *"The literature demonstrates clearly negative impacts of aluminum on the nervous system across the age span."*[15]

The authors of the study observed a potential link between aluminum and autism:

> *"In young children, a highly significant correlation exists between the number of pediatric aluminum-adjuvanted vaccines administered and the rate of autism spectrum disorders."*[16]

In 2011, Shoenfeld and Agmon-Levin published a paper suggesting that certain autoimmune or autoinflammatory symptoms were so similar in both conditions—and they also appeared to result from the adjuvant in the vaccine—they suggested use of the umbrella term: Autoimmune/inflammatory Syndrome Induced by Adjuvants (ASIA).[17] In 2016 they wrote a paper continuing the subject by adding to their research into how thyroid or "endocrine autoimmune diseases can be triggered by adjuvants, configuring cases of ASIA syndrome."[18]

Doctors and other health professionals are starting to acknowledge this new umbrella term and its relationship to vaccine injuries.

Another research paper[19] talks about a condition called Macrophagic myofasciitis (MMF or MF), a disorder that seems to be rapidly increasing. It falls under the umbrella of ASIA, along with illnesses such as the Gulf War Syndrome (GWS) and siliconosis.

On the World Health Organization's (WHO) website is an article stating that research has shown aluminum-containing vaccines could be the cause of MMF[20].

Other aluminum-associated disorders include lupus, diabetes, Alzheimer's disease (AD), arthritis, Hashimoto's, Guillain-Barré syndrome (GBS) and many others. We investigate some of them in more depth in future chapters.

Chapter 9: Aluminum, it's getting on my cells

[1] Kawahara, M. and Kato-Negishi, M. (2011). Link between Aluminum and the Pathogenesis of Alzheimer's Disease: The Integration of the Aluminum and Amyloid Cascade Hypotheses. *Int J Alzheimers Dis*, 2011, 276393

[2] Keele University. (n.d.). *Professor Chris Exley*. Retrieved from www.keele.ac.uk/aluminium/groupmembers/chrisexley/

[3] Keele University. (n.d.). *Professor Chris Exley*. Retrieved from www.keele.ac.uk/aluminium/groupmembers/chrisexley/

[4] Keele University. (n.d.). *Professor Chris Exley Publications*. Retrieved from www.keele.ac.uk/aluminium/groupmembers/chrisexley/publications/

[5] The Hippocratic Post. (n.d.). *About Us*. Retrieved from www.hippocraticpost.com/about-us/

[6] Exley, C. (2007, November 30). *Aluminium and autism*. Retrieved from www.hippocraticpost.com/infection-disease/aluminium-and-autism/

[7] Mold, M., Umar, D., King, A., and Exley, C. (2018). Aluminium in brain tissue in autism. *Journal of Trace Elements in Medicine and Biology*, 46, 76-82 www.doi.org/10.1016/j.jtemb.2017.11.012

[8] Exley, C. (2007, November 30). *Aluminium and autism*. Retrieved from www.hippocraticpost.com/infection-disease/aluminium-and-autism/

[9] HogenEsch, H. (2012). Mechanism of Immunopotentiation and Safety of Aluminum Adjuvants. *Front Immunol*, 3, 406

[10] National Kidney Foundation. (n.d.). *Glomerular Filtration Rate (GFR)*. Retrieved from www.kidney.org/atoz/content/gfr

[11] Shaw C.A., Seneff, S., Kette, S.D., Tomljenovic, L., Oller Jr., J.W., and Davidson, R.M. (2014). Aluminum-Induced Entropy in Biological Systems: Implications for Neurological Disease. *Journal of Toxicology*, 2014, 491316.

[12] Ibid.

[13] Ibid.

[14] Tomljenovic, L. and Shaw C. (2011).Aluminum vaccine adjuvants: are they safe? *Curr Med Chem*, 18(17), 2630-2637.

[15] Shaw C., and Tomljenovic L. (2013). Aluminum in the central nervous system (CNS): toxicity in humans and animals, vaccine adjuvants, and autoimmunity. *Immunologic Research*, 56(2-3), 304-316.

[16] Ibid.

[17] Shoenfeld, Y., and Agmon-Levin, N. (2011). Autoimmuni/inflammatory syndrome induced by adjuvants. *J Autoimmun*, 36(1), 4-8.

[18] Watad, A., David, A., Brown, S., and Shoenfeld, Y. (2016). Autoimmune/Inflammatory Syndrome Induced by Adjuvants and Thyroid Autoimmunity. *Front Endocrinol (Lausanne)*, 7, 150.

[19] Couette M., Boisse, M.F., Maison, P., Brugieres, P., Cesaro, P., Chevalier, X., ... Authier, F.J. (2009). Long-term persistence of vaccine-derived aluminum hydroxide is associated with chronic cognitive dysfunction. *Journal of Inorganic Biochemistry*, 103(11), 1571-1578.

---

[20] The World Health Organization. (n.d.). *Macrophagic myofasciitis and aluminium-containing vaccines.* Retrieved from
www.who.int/vaccine_safety/committee/reports/october_1999/en/

CHAPTER 10

Aluminum controversy

"I have discovered with advancing years that
few things are entirely black or white, but more
often different shades of grey."

~*Jeffrey Archer,* A Prisoner of Birth

The Aluminum (Al) conundrum is an entire rabbit hole on its own and it's beyond us why this neurotoxic adjuvant is still being used in vaccines.

It's very difficult to pinpoint concerns to specific vaccines when an ingredient used in multiple vaccines may be the culprit. Not only that, it could be that the ingredient is the straw that breaks the camel's back, so to speak, after a child's body is or has been fighting many other chemicals in their food and environment.

Dr. Paul Offit, with the *Children's Hospital of Philadelphia*[1], a leading advocate for childhood vaccines and co-developer of the rotavirus vaccine in America, doesn't feel there is cause for concern. He states:

> *"No, aluminum shouldn't be concerning to parents because the quantities of aluminum that are in vaccines, again, are trivial."*[2]

The quote was taken from a phone interview transcript with *Sound Advice* run by *American Academy of Pediatrics*[3]. Dr. Offit continues:

> *"Aluminum salts are used in vaccines and frankly, have been used in vaccines since the 1940s as something called an adjuvant, and what an adjuvant means is it actually enhances the immune response."*[4]

There have been countless studies since the 1940s showing an obvious link between neurological damage and aluminum, and we have already named a few. Surely they can't all be wrong?

Dr. Offit adds:

> *"Aluminum at very high levels can be toxic, but when it is toxic, it's toxic really only in two circumstances. [...] One is a child whose kidneys don't work who is also receiving high quantities of aluminum in the intravenous fluids that they're receiving or in antacids. [...] aluminum is toxic only in those settings."*[5]

So, unless you are a child in kidney failure, receiving aluminum IV or eating antacids, you are good to go. Or maybe not? We suspect not.

One more question. How much aluminum is there in a vaccine?

Dr. Offit continues:

> *"People tend to generally ingest between five to 10 milligrams of aluminum a day, [...] and the quantity that's in vaccines is measured in the microgram level, [...] So again, just in terms of scale, the quantity of aluminum that you're exposed to in vaccines is much, much less than you would be exposed to if you, for example, ate a pancake."*[6]

Are the trace amounts of aluminum really nothing to worry about? As Dr. Offit said, we are ingesting so much more in our daily food than we get from a vaccine. We find this a little confusing.

There is enough aluminum in the vaccine to aggravate our immune system to the point it tricks our cells into thinking we have a living germ invading our body. In fact, the body starts attacking the dead or dissected germ. Yet, somehow, the aluminum is not strong enough to damage our cells?

Digest, inject & eject

Any aluminum we (unknowingly?) digest when eating is not absorbed very well. According to Dr. Exley, "[t]he body burden of aluminum is a dynamic entity" and depends on its individual, so measuring how much aluminum is excreted is difficult to calculate. In his paper published on the *Royal Society of Chemistry* website, he adds a very clear image of aluminum route of entry and exit in relation to the human body. He explains that aluminum is excreted "by a number of routes including *via* the faeces, urine, sweat, skin, hair, nails, sebum and semen." It is therefore impossible to measure a standard amount of aluminum excreted for all individuals. Dr. Exley gives an example by sharing a study done in the 80s where fecal excretion of aluminum ranged "between 74 and 96% of the ingested amount"[7].

Regardless of how little is left in the body, even if less than a percentage, is what the remaining aluminum circulating in the blood stream does to our body. This, of course, is dependent on our health and on what other medications or products are also in the body. It's also important to note that the bloodstream leads straight to our organs, including the brain.

Luckily for us, the bloodstream takes the aluminum to our kidneys. If they are healthy, they're great at eliminating toxins. So, most of the remaining aluminum passes through the kidneys. It's obviously difficult to assess the overall damage incurred in this process because as you can see, much depends on the health of the individual.

Blood-brain barrier

Protecting our brain from foreign substances is the blood-brain barrier (BBB). This barrier protects our brain and spinal cord. Apart from problems resulting from an immature, aged or diseased blood-brain barrier, there are many toxins that can damage it—aluminum and mercury included.

One way aluminum (Al) can penetrate the blood brain barrier is by hiding in Trojan horse-like fashion inside a macrophage (Mφ). As discussed earlier, the macrophages (phagocytes) eat the invading particles that are covered with aluminum. The macrophages then travel up the bloodstream to the lymph nodes where our T cells and B cells are hanging out. This is also the same route as to all the organs, including the brain. It just so happens the macrophages are capable of crossing the blood-brain barrier delivering aluminum to the brain.

Dosage

A paper on Alzheimer's disease (AD) from 2010, mentioned earlier in the chapter, says:

> *"According to the latest vaccination schedule, every child in the USA will receive a total of 5–6 mg of Al by the age of 2 years, or up to 1.475 mg of Al during a single visit to the pediatrician."*[8]

We wondered what the US Food and Drug Administration (FDA) feels about this. Title 21 of the Code of Federal Regulations says:

> *"An adjuvant shall not be introduced into a product unless there is satisfactory evidence that it does not affect adversely the safety or potency of the product. The amount of aluminum in the recommended individual dose of a biological product shall not exceed:*
>
> *"(1) 0.85 milligrams if determined by assay;*
>
> *"(2) 1.14 milligrams if determined by calculation on the basis of the amount of aluminum compound added; or*
>
> *"(3) 1.25 milligrams determined by assay provided that data demonstrating that the amount of aluminum used is safe and necessary to produce the intended effect [...]."*[9]

What the FDA fails to include is whether it's okay to inject multiple vaccines simultaneously. Nonetheless, the amounts of aluminum a child receives in a doctor's visit, as mentioned above, is still higher than the limits stated in the FDA's Title 21.

Site of injection

The vaccine needle-stick can also cause a slight trauma at the stick location. Toxins that are at the site and not transported away from it can cause the area to become inflamed. The body's immune cells are fighting hard against these aluminum-coated antigens.

There's a possibility these adjuvant-coated antigens attach themselves to our own cells. Among others, these include nerve cells, muscle cells or platelets even.

As you now know, some immune cells are tasked with gathering and delivering information about the invader. When, for instance, B cells receive this information, they start pumping out a vast amount of antibodies. And when antibodies find foreign objects that match the information they were programmed with, they latch on to these objects.

When these foreign objects are attached to our own cells, antibodies may not be able to recognize they are actually our own cells and latch on to them as if they were foreign. In other words, this tricks B cells into creating antibodies against the body's own cells and thereby cause an autoimmune response.

Chapter 10: Aluminum controversy

[1] Wikipedia. (2018, October 15). *Paul Offit*. Retrieved from www.en.wikipedia.org/wiki/Paul_Offit

[2] American Academy of Pediatrics. (2009, April). *Sound Advice*. [transcript of a telephone interview]. Retrieved from www.healthychildren.org/English/sa fety-prevention/immunizations/Documents/Offit-Transcript.pdf

[3] American Academy of Pediatrics. (2018). *Healthy Children*. Retrieved from www.healthychildren.org/English/Pages/default.aspx

[4] Ibid.

[5] Ibid.

[6] Ibid.

[7] Exley, C. (2013) Human exposure to aluminum. *Environ. Scie.: Processes Impacts*, 15: 1807-1816

[8] Tomljenovic, L. (2013). Aluminum and Alzheimer's Disease:After a Century of Controversy,Is there a Plausible Link?. *Journal of Alzheimer's Disease*, 23(4), 567-598.

[9] U.S. Food and Drug Administration. (2018, April 1). *CFR - Code of Federal Regulations Title 21*. Retrieved from www.accessdata.fda.gov/scripts/cdrh/cfdocs/cfcfr/CFRSearch.cfm?fr=610.15

CHAPTER 11

Definitely maybe science

"The signature of mediocrity is not an unwillingness to change. The signature of mediocrity is inconsistency."

~James C. Collins (American author and lecturer).

When reviewing multiple papers on the same topic, we have noticed it's quite common to find inconsistencies in the observations recorded. Research that should be reproducible and therefore consistent regardless of which scientists are performing it, appears to diminish the closer we look.

A research paper on the effects of aluminum in Alzheimer's disease (AD) from 2011 states:

> *"Whilst being environmentally abundant, aluminum is not essential for life. On the contrary, aluminum is widely recognized neurotoxin that inhibits more than 200 biologically important functions and causes various adverse effects in plants, animals and humans."* [1]

A Dr. Thomas Jefferson[2] was "funded to investigate vaccine safety by the European Commission,"[3] and was at the time "the head of the vaccine division of the Cochrane Collaboration"[4].

This collaboration has as of December 7th, 2018:

> *"13,000 members and over 50,000 supporters come from more than 130 countries, worldwide. Our volunteers and contributors are researchers, health professionals, patients, carers, and people passionate about improving health outcomes for everyone, everywhere. Our global*

independent network gathers and summarizes the best evidence from research to help you make informed choices about treatment [...].

"We do not accept commercial or conflicted funding. This is vital for us to generate authoritative and reliable information, working freely, unconstrained by commercial and financial interests."[5]

In a research paper on aluminum in diphtheria, tetanus and pertussis (DTP) vaccines from 2004, Dr. Jefferson states that:

"We found no evidence that aluminium salts in vaccines cause any serious or long-lasting adverse events. Despite a lack of good-quality evidence we do not recommend that any further research on this topic is undertaken." [6]

Confused? We were a little perplexed, so we looked for any commentary regarding this paper. We found a petition from 2014 requesting the retraction of this paper[78]. To the best of our knowledge, the paper still has not been retracted as of publication of this book.

Elizabeth Hart[9], the petitioner, continues using the authors own words where they state "[o]verall, the methodological quality of included studies was low."[10] She continues by using Dr. Jefferson's own conclusion in his paper:

"Data has enabled us to reach firm conclusions on the limited amount of comparative data available. [...] The results of our review should be interpreted within the limited quantity and quality of available evidence."[11]

To help validate her argument, she continues to use Dr. Jefferson's own words, this time from 2002 where he states that:

"Most safety studies on childhood vaccines have not been conducted thoroughly enough to tell whether the jabs cause side effects. [...] There is some good research, but it is overwhelmed by the bad. The public has been let down because the proper studies have not been done."[12]

We understand her argument and feel our notion on the studies' lack of weight has been validated. The authors are suggesting we can actually make scientifically *firm conclusions* on *limited data?*

There are *firm conclusions* on *limited quantity and quality data* that should be *interpreted within* those limits.

Let's recap: A study with limited and low-quality data was able to arrive at such definitive conclusions that there's no need to do any more research into this topic.

Hart wasn't the only one putting this research review under scrutiny. Another review was performed by the University of York which is:

> "*a dynamic, research-intensive university committed to the development of life-saving discoveries and new technologies to tackle some of the most pressing global challenges.*"[13]

The University of York's Centre for Reviews and Dissemination (CRD) finds the data and methods used for Jefferson's study were appropriately collected and that:

> "*The quality of studies was assessed and the findings of the review were discussed in the context of the poor quality evidence available. The analysis seemed appropriate, albeit restricted by the small numbers of studies included.*
>
> "*The authors' conclusions seem reasonable, but the limited quantity and poor quality of the evidence on which they are based should be kept in mind.*"[14]
>
> *We were curious to see whether Dr. Jefferson was still the head of the Cochrane*

Collaboration's vaccine division, so we visited Cochrane's webpage and were able to confirm he was, or is, still with the collaboration.

However, an announcement on the site caught our eye. Headlined *Closure of the Vaccine Field,* and reads as follows:

> "*The Cochrane Vaccine Field has ceased operation effective 1 November 2015. An ongoing lack of resource capacity meant that the team were unable to continue to provide a coordinating base and we thank them for all of their hard work.*"[15]

From the above research, we know *the Cochrane Collaboration* has been studying effects of vaccines at least since 2004. More than a decade later, in 2015, they felt they didn't have enough information to continue reviewing the safety of vaccines. It's difficult to comprehend that due to inefficient data and lack of resources, they were forced to end their research into vaccine safety.

Dr. Jefferson explains why the aluminum adjuvant is not being withdrawn and replaced:

> *"Assessment of the safety of aluminum in vaccines is important because replacement of aluminum compounds in currently licensed vaccines would necessitate the introduction of a completely new compound that would have to be investigated before licensing. No obvious candidates to replace aluminum are available, so withdrawal for safety reasons would severely affect the immunogenicity and protective effects of some currently licensed vaccines and threaten immunization programs worldwide."*[16]

When a group like *the Cochrane Collaboration* is unable to find enough studies with reliable data being conducted worldwide on vaccines, it must be said we have a serious problem in the scientific vaccine research community.

We can't help but ask the question: why? Why is there not enough reliable data? And since there isn't enough reliable data, why did Cochrane's vaccine division shut down? Is that not a concern?

It appears the more questions we ask ourselves, the more confused we become about the ambiguity in the vaccine field.

Aluminum didn't have to go through any rigorous testing because it was implemented *before* the current adjuvant regulations took effect.

So far other adjuvants, which are being studied *after* the adjuvant regulation took effect, have failed to be as effective as aluminum, and therefore scientists haven't been able to find a replacement adjuvant. However, we must wonder, if aluminum were to be compared, using the same standards as we have today, would it still do better than its potential competing adjuvants?

If, let's say a different adjuvant had been used first, before the current regulations were introduced, and aluminum was being researched under the regulations implemented today, would it be approved?

It's in your head

There was a very interesting study done in the 1990s that we feel hasn't gotten the recognition it deserves. It was released in *PubMed* in 2010[17] some 10 years after it was conducted. Now two decades since the study was done, as far as we can tell, discussions about this study and its results are almost non-existent.

The study we refer to randomly selected 16 infant rhesus monkeys and divided them into two groups. One group of 12 infant monkeys received the 1990's CDC's recommended childhood vaccine schedule at the same rate children in the US would. The remaining four infant monkeys, which comprised the control group, received placebo (saline) vaccines according to the same schedule. (It would be interesting if they added a second control group using the placebos used in vaccine safety studies today. We are very curious to know how it would compare).

This was a longitudinal study lasting from 1994 to 1999 to follow the vaccine schedule in a proper timeline. The study found the vaccinated monkeys had a much "greater total brain volume" than the average healthy brain. They also observed that the amygdala in the vaccinated monkeys didn't mature with time as it was supposed to. The amygdala, incidentally, plays an important role in social interactions.

Maybe it's not so surprising they also observed that in the vaccinated monkeys the opioid antagonist diprenorphine (DPN) levels never lowered throughout the study. In the placebo group, the DPN levels decreased noticeably. One function of DPN is to block social interaction. What this means is the research showed that the social behavior of those monkeys that received the actual vaccines, where the DPN levels did not decrease, turned anti-social.

We found there was at least one more study undertaken to verify the association between DPN and social behavior. Performed in 1981[18]. The authors of that study believe the release of opioids in the brain encourages social interactions. So, when the body fails to decrease the amount of the antagonist DPN, it not only blocks the opioids that encourage social interactions, but it blocks the *desire* to socially interact.

We were unable to find published studies that show a link between DPN and autism. *However,* we did look a little closer into DPN. Apparently, there are three different variations of opioid receptors: mu, μ; delta, δ; and kappa, κ.[19] We are only interested in the kappa (κ1 and κ2) receptors. There are more kappa receptors in the brain than any other opioid receptor. Not surprisingly, you'll find these receptors in the amygdala.[20] The paper states:

> *"The κ opioid receptors have been implicated in several clinical brain disorders, including drug abuse, epilepsy, Tourette's syndrome, and Alzheimer's disease."*[21]

What DPN does is bind to the kappa receptors and that's how it accumulates in the amygdala. So, it makes sense how DPN could cause problems when it doesn't go away with time.

We came across another study that found a correlation between an abnormal amygdala and neurological dysfunctions. If you recall, the amygdala in the monkeys receiving the true vaccines failed to mature. The study supports the view that the amygdala plays an important role in social interactions and has "been implicated in numerous neuropsychiatric and neurodevelopmental disorders."[22]

As explained in a study from 2018, the amygdala plays "a critical role in fear, emotion, and social behavior."[23] This research study evaluated brains of "24 neurotypical and 28 autism spectrum disorder (ASD)" individuals between the ages two and 48. Regarding ASD and the size of the amygdala, the authors state:

> *"Alterations in amygdala growth can be detected as early as 2 y of age and persist into late childhood. The severity of the individual's social and communicative symptoms positively correlates with amygdala enlargement, suggesting a potential structure–function relationship."*[24]

What the authors also found is that in a neurotypical brain, the number of mature nerve cells increased with time, while in the brain of ASD individuals, the "number of mature neurons" appeared to decrease with time.

Another study posted on Stanford University School of Medicine's website shows that the size of the amygdala correlates with a child's anxiety level. The bigger the amygdala, the higher the anxiety level.[25]

In yet another study into the amygdala in children, it was shown that children with autism had an enlarged amygdala compared to children without autism[26].

Also, a study into Alzheimer's disease (AD) from 2010, mentions accumulation of the adjuvant aluminum (Al) in, among other places, the amygdala.[27]

This got us thinking, since autistic individuals have been shown to have abnormal amygdalae, perhaps there is also aluminum on the amygdala in children with autism.

Unfortunately, we couldn't find studies that tested the presence of aluminum in the amygdala of children with autism or enlarged amygdala.

Scientists may not know exactly which parts of the vaccines our body decides to react to. Each person reacts so differently. But it seems likely there is validity in questioning vaccine safety when a concoction of substances is used to provoke our immune system.

Because each immune system is different, scientists can't predict its reaction when presented with something foreign. Especially when the vaccine contains scientifically proven neurotoxins, such as aluminum.

Chapter 11: Definitely maybe science

[1] Kawahara, M. and Kato-Negishi, M. (2011). Link between Aluminum and the Pathogenesis of Alzheimer's Disease: The Integration of the Aluminum and Amyloid Cascade Hypotheses. *Int J Alzheimers Dis*, 2011, 276393

[2] Cochrane Nordic. (2018). *Tom Jefferson*. Retrieved from www.nordic.cochrane.org/tom-jefferson

[3] Fraser, L. (2002, October 27). *Vaccines expert warns studies are useless*. Retrieved from www.telegraph.co.uk/news/uknews/1411417/Vaccines-expert-warns-studies-are-useless.html

[4] Ibid.

[5] Cochrane. (n.d.). *About us*. Retrieved from www.cochrane.org/about-us

[6] Jefferson, T., Rudin, M., and Pietrantonj, C.D. (2004). Adverse events after immunisation with aluminium-containing DTP vaccines: systematic review of the evidence. *The Lancet*, 4(2), 84-90

[7] Hart, E. (2014, July 8). [Letter to Professor Gotzche]. Retrieved from www.users.on.net/~peter.hart/Challenge_to_Cochrane_re_vax-safety_and_aluminium.pdf

[8] Hart, E. (2014, July 17). [Letter to Professor Gotzche]. Retrieved from www.users.on.net/~peter.hart/Vaccine_safety_and_aluminium_follow-up_to_Cochrane.pdf

[9] Hart, E. (n.d.). *About Elizabeth Hart*. [Web log post]. Retrieved from www.over-vaccination.net/about-2/

[10] Hart, E. (2014, July 8). *Vaccine safety and aluminium – a challenge to The Cochrane Collaboration*. Retrieved from www.over-vaccination.net/tag/bexsero/

[11] Ibid.

[12] Ibid.

[13] University of York. (n.d.). *About the University*. Retrieved from www.york.ac.uk/about/

[14] Jefferson, T., Rudin, M., and Di, P.C., (n.d.). *Adverse events after immunisation with aluminium-containing DTP vaccines: systematic review of the evidence*. Retrieved from www.crd.york.ac.uk/crdweb/ShowRecord.asp?LinkFrom=OAI&ID=12004000414

[15] Cochrane Community. (2015, November 18). *Closure of the Vaccines Field*. Retrieved from www.community.cochrane.org/news/closure-vaccines-field

[16] Humphries, S. (2015, February 24). Dr Suzanne Humphries. *Aluminum is toxic to all life forms: The case against aluminum in vaccines* (Location in video: 31:18). [Video link]. Retrieved from www.youtube.com/watch?v=LZe99K12740

[17] Hewitson, L., Lopresti, B.J., Stott, C., Mason, N.S., and Tomko, J. (2010). Influence of pediatric vaccines on amygdala growth and opioid ligand binding in rhesus macaque infants: A pilot study. *Acta Neurobiol Exp*, 70(2), 147-164

[18] Panksepp, B. and Bishop, P. (1981). An autoradiographic map of (3H) diprenorphine binding in rat brain: Effects of social interaction. *Brain Research Bulletin*, 7(4), 405-410.

[19] Leung K. [6-O-methyl-11C]Diprenorphine. (2006 May 24). [Updated 2007 May 12]. In: Molecular Imaging and Contrast Agent Database (MICAD) [Internet]. Bethesda (MD): National Center for Biotechnology Information (US); 2004-2013. Available from: https://www.ncbi.nlm.nih.gov/books/NBK23399/

[20] Ibid.

[21] Ibid.

[22] Schumann, C.M., Bauman, M.D., and Amaral, D.G. (2010). Abnormal structure or function of the amygdala is a common component of neurodevelopmental disorders. *Neuropsychologia*, 49(4), 745-759.

[23] Avino, T. A., Barger, N., Vargas, M. V., Carlson, E. L., Amaral, D. G., Bauman, M. D., & Schumann, C. M. (2018). Neuron numbers increase in the human amygdala from birth to adulthood, but not in autism. *Proceedings of the National Academy of Sciences of the United States of America*, 115(14), 3710-3715.

[24] Ibid.

[25] Stanford University. (2013, November 20). *Size, connectivity of brain region linked to anxiety level in young children, study shows*. Retrieved from www.med.stanford.edu/news/all-news/2013/11/size-connectivity-of-brain-region-linked-to-anxiety-level-in-young-children-study-shows.html

[26] Schuman, C.M, Hamstra, J., Goodlin-Jones, B.L., Lotspeich, L.J., Kwon, H., Buonocore, M.H., ... Amaral, D.G. (2004). The Amygdala Is Enlarged in Children But Not Adolescents with Autism; the Hippocampus Is Enlarged at All Ages. *Journal of Neuroscience*, 24(28), 6392-6401.

[27] Tomljenovic, L. (2011). Aluminum and Alzheimer's Disease: After a Century of Controversy, Is there a Plausible Link?. *Journal of Alzheimer's Disease*, 23(4): 567-598.

CHAPTER 12

Formaldehyde—The demolition crew

"To alcohol! The cause of... and solution to...
all of life's problems"

~Matt Groening (American cartoonist)

When scientists use the entire germ in the vaccine, they have to kill it or weaken it substantially before putting it into the vaccine. In order to do this, they use a chemical. The most common chemical for this process is Formaldehyde (FA) or Formalin (liquid form of formaldehyde).

Many scientists have expressed concern about injecting embalming fluid into the bodies of little infants. We thought therefore we should take a closer look at the validity of this concern. In order to do this, we need to know which part of our body it affects and what formaldehyde does when directly exposed to our cells.

When formaldehyde comes in direct contact with our cells, it compromises the integrity of the tau proteins inside the cells. Nerve cells have the most tau proteins out of all the cells, so they are the most vulnerable.

Just like humans, each cell has a skeleton called cytoskeleton (which literally means cell-skeleton). The main component of a cytoskeleton is the microtubules. These tubules are made up of thousands of paired-up proteins. A protein-pair has one alpha and one beta tubulin. They always go together, two and two, as alpha and beta. When assembled, they form a spiral called microtubules. It looks a lot like a pearl necklace wrapped around a tube.

This structure can't be built without help. The alpha and beta tubulins need to be tied together in order to stabilize. Our cells use tau proteins to do this. Because these microtubular structures are made up of thousands of tiny tubulins, they are quite flexible.

The way the tau proteins bind the alpha and beta subunits together allows the microtubules to assemble, disassemble and reassemble, grow and shrink as needed at any given time.

When they disassemble, the tau proteins let go of each alpha and beta subunit. The tubulins will disburse inside the cell and float around until called to duty. When signaled, tau proteins will reassemble them as commanded. This means the body is constantly building microtubular structures then tearing them down and rebuilding them. This constant construction is happening inside all our cells at any given moment in time. Without it, the cell would not function.

You may be wondering why there's a need to worry so much about formaldehyde messing with the tau proteins when it's a structural thing. It's not like it's destroying the function of the cell, right? Let's take a closer look.

It's a jungle in here

Many would probably define the human skeleton as something like supportive columns and compare it to steel beams on a skyscraper or poles in a tent. However, our cells are more complex than that and need the skeleton to serve multiple purposes.

Before we continue, we'd like to remind you that we have different cells in our bodies, so our explanation here relates to that of a general cell. The same occurrence within a nerve cell would be described a little differently, but the concept is the same.

Let's say you live in a hut near the center of a vast jungle. Inside our cellular *jungle,* we call this hut the Centrosome, which sits next to the nucleus inside the cell. The cellular *jungle* contains a lot of *inhabitants* who need a ride to get from place to place. These *inhabitants* are generally referred to as *cargo.*[1]

In order to transport this cellular cargo, there's a vast network of microtubules in place. To continue using our jungle analogy, this would be like a vast network of ziplines. The ziplines being the microtubules. These ziplines are used for transportation of cargo both near and far, inside the cell. The microtubules are charged, with the minus end towards the inner part of the cell and the plus end towards the outer part of cell.

In order for transportation to take place, there needs to be a way to attach the cargo on to the zipline or microtubules. This is done by using a motor protein which serves as a buckle of some sort. When the cargo is being transported in the plus direction (towards outer part of the cell), this motor protein is called kinesin. When the transport is going in the minus direction (towards the inner part of cell), it uses a protein called dynein. (A third motor protein used in muscle contraction is called myosin). In a nerve cell the microtubules would be travelling along the axon. Considering the fact that kinesin travels outward, on a nerve cell that means it travels away from nucleus and down the axon. The dynein would be traveling towards the dendrites. [2]

The cell also uses the ziplines to get information out to the surface of the cell in order to communicate with other cells and the *outside world*. Unfortunately, it's not just our own cellular components that take advantage of this fantastic communication and transportation network. Some viruses also take advantage and utilize the microtubules for their own purposes.[3] We won't go into more detail on that, just something to keep in mind.

When the microtubules perform their various important functions, the tau proteins (the support ties) can change the way your genes are being expressed.[4] They help protect your DNA and possibly help repair it as well.[5]

So far, we have established that microtubules serve as support columns to provide structure/support and as a vast network of ziplines for transportation/communication inside the cell. Another cool microtubule feature is, as the name implies, it's also hollow on the inside.

Inside our cells we have an immense amount of proteins. Some of these proteins have specific tasks or messages they need to transport to other locations in the cell. So, the proteins will latch on to the kinesin or dynein (buckle) on the zipline to catch a ride. As mentioned, the cable is hollow, which means there's something going on in the *tunnels* or inside the microtubules. Yes, our cells have their very own underground network. [6]

Another important task the microtubules are a part of, is separating the chromosomes during cell division. This is where the motor proteins myosin are used. They anchor the chromosomes down then flex to become shorter, meaning the tau proteins remove some of the alpha and beta subunits in order to shorten. This pulls the chromosomes apart. And voila! There you have it. Cell division!

Movin' to the groovin'

As we explained, the microtubules are extremely important in dividing cells and moving things around inside cells. But this isn't all they do. The microtubules also move the entire cell around.

Cilia, which are hair-like structures on the surface of the cell, are actually microtubules.

The cell uses the cilia to move around by either moving itself or the fluid around it. Then there are some cells that have flagella. These can look like long tails on the cell, but are actually just a bunch of microtubules. They work more like a motor, propelling the cell around.

Many parts of our bodies have cilia. Some cilia move around while others don't, being more for sensory purposes. These sensory cilia are located in places such as the kidneys and eyes. In the eyes, the cilia move the signals from one cell to another.

The cilia that moves around, is found, for instance, in the respiratory tract where it's used to transfer mucus and other particles away from the lungs and out of the body. This is also how the Fallopian tubes move the egg. When it comes to the flagella, an example would be how it steers the sperm toward the egg.

In the brain we have nerve cells or neurons. The microtubules in these cells are also extremely important in communication between nerve cells in the brain.

As you can see, the tau proteins are quite busy making life possible (for us). When something goes wrong with the tau proteins, where their ability to tie the alpha and beta subunits together has failed, the microtubules will fall apart. When this happens, the cells are unable to move things around. Instead, the microtubules become tangled up inside the cell. This destroys the cell. Formaldehyde (FA) can cause this to happen in as little as 0.01–0.1% FA solution.[7]

How does this amount of formaldehyde compare to that in vaccines?

Chapter 12: Formaldehyde – The demolition crew

[1] Balabanian, L., Chaudhary, A.R., and Hendricks, A.G. (2018). Traffic control inside the cell: microtubule-based regulation of cargo transport. *Biochemical Society*, 40(2), 14-17.

[2] Franker, M.A.M. and Hoogenraad, C.C. (2013). Microtubule-based transport – basic mechanisms, traffic rules and role in neurological pathogenesis. *Journal of Cell Science*, 126, 1-11.

[3] Niehl, A., Pena, E.J., Amari, K., and Heinlein, M. (2013). Microtubules in viral replication and transport. *The Plant Journal*, 75, 290-308.

[4] Sultan, A., Nesslany, F., Violet, M., Bégard, S., Loyens, A., Talahari, S., Mansuroglu, Z., Marzin, D., Sergeant, N., Humez, S., Colin, M., Bonnefoy, E., Buée, L., … Galas, M. C. (2010). Nuclear tau, a key player in neuronal DNA protection. *The Journal of biological chemistry*, 286(6), 4566-4575.

[5] Guo, T., Noble, W. and Hanger, D.P. (2017). Roles of Tau Protein in Health and Disease. *Acta Neuropathologica*, 133(5): 665–704.

[6] The Protein Experts. (2013, May). *Life Inside a Microtubule*. Retrieved from www.cytoskeleton.com/pdf-storage/news/life-inside-a-microtubule.pdf

[7] Ibid.

CHAPTER 13

The right amount

*"I was not allowed to take spherical
trigonometry because I'd sprained my ankle.
Because I'd sprained my ankle, I had an
incomplete in gym, phys ed. And the rule was
that if you had an incomplete in anything, you
were not allowed to take an overload."*

~**William Shockley** *(American physicist).*

In certain vaccines, formaldehyde (FA) is used to "inactivate viruses and to detoxify bacterial toxins."[1] In the making of a vaccine almost all the toxins are eliminated. Unfortunately, it's impossible to extract all the toxins. There will always be some residual toxins left in the vaccine. When it comes to formaldehyde, this can be 0.02% FA or less.

As with other chemicals, the various forms should not be confused. We mentioned in the previous chapter that formaldehyde becomes formalin when in liquid. To be more specific, when methyl alcohol is added to formaldehyde, it becomes formalin. A solution that's 10% formalin, is actually 3.7–4% formaldehyde.[2]

In the above-referenced study the authors compared "formaldehyde-containing vaccines at a single medical visit" to the natural occurring formaldehyde levels "in a model 2-month-old infant." The results were:

> *"[...] a single dose of 200 µg, formaldehyde is essentially completely removed from the site of injection within 30 min."* [3]

This study concludes that the injected "formaldehyde continues to be safe." [4] Another study, using the same low formaldehyde (FA) solution states that "the presence of formaldehyde" causes tau proteins to aggregate and "become inactive in tubulin assembly."[5] So, even at low levels formaldehyde changes tau's integrity.

Another study shows that a very small amount of formaldehyde solution is needed to cause accumulation of amyloid-beta proteins.[6] When these proteins accumulate in the hippocampus, they become larger and toxic to neurons. Hippocampus deals for the most part with short-term, long-term and spatial memory. When cells die, the brain loses various functions and memory loss is inevitable.[7]

During our research digging we found it difficult to understand how so many scientific studies out there can be studying the exact same thing, yet their conclusions completely contradict each other. Formaldehyde studies are no exception. If each study can be replicated by a third party in the laboratory, how can the results vary so greatly?

Our body produces formaldehyde naturally. This makes it difficult to determine how safe formaldehyde in vaccines really is. Formaldehyde can damage our cells, but at the same time it can defend the cells against damage. In the latter case, our body breaks the formaldehyde down into smaller pieces. These smaller pieces are no longer formaldehyde, but are now formate.[8] The cell uses formate to create more DNA.

Normally our cells are destroyed by being broken apart. Formaldehyde doesn't do that. As you may know, each cell has multiple proteins on its surface. These surface proteins serve as communicators between cells and between the cell and its surrounding environment. Formaldehyde crosslinks these surface proteins together, so the cells can't communicate properly with each other or their environment.

This is exactly why formaldehyde is used in vaccines, to kill or inactivate the vaccine germs and contaminants during production phase: by crosslinking the proteins on the cell surface.[910]

Some health professionals are concerned about formaldehyde accumulating in the body. For example, Sherri Tenpenny, Doctor of Osteopathic Medicine (DO), who has great insight into the field of natural health, argues that by the time a child is five, they have received 1.795 mg Formaldehyde.

Dr. Tenpenny says:

> *"Through sloppy and negligent math, lawmakers and manufacturers fail to throw up a red flag regarding the*

*large amount of formaldehyde injected into young bodies
with developing brains, neurological systems and
organs."[11]*

So why is it that so many health professionals show no concern for
formaldehyde safety in vaccines? Could it be that it's because it has a short
lifespan and the body's natural ability to take care of it is already in place?

The normal levels of formaldehyde in our blood is about 2.5 mg/l.
Formaldehyde is only active for about 1.5 minutes in the body. Using this
to calculate, the conclusion will be that "an adult human liver will
metabolize 22 mg formaldehyde per minute." This metabolized
formaldehyde then becomes carbon dioxide and pushed out of the
body.[12]

A research paper from The University of Queensland Brain Institute
in Australia did studies on formaldehyde damage on the cell. They used
three different concentrations of formaldehyde: 0.1 mmol/l, 0.2 mmol/l
and 0.3 mmol/l. So as not to confuse units together, we converted them
to mg/l units.[13] When they tested the mice with 3.0 mg/l (0.1 mmol/l)
and 6.0 mg/l (0.2 mmol/l), they noticed the damage blocked cell division,
while a concentration of 9.0 mg/l (0.3 mmol/l) completely destroyed the
cell.[14]

If we assume an adult body has five liters of blood and a child's body
half that[15], using Children's Hospital of Philadelphia's (CHOP) example,
a two-month-old infant, weighing 5 kg has 1.1 mg circulating in the blood
at any given time.[16]

Using their list of vaccines containing formaldehyde and calculating
the combined formaldehyde content in the vaccine schedule for a two-
month-old infant, which is DTaP, Polio and Hepatitis B, assuming max
amounts, we get about 0.2 mg formaldehyde.[17]

There you have it. Nothing to be concerned about, right?

The amount of formaldehyde in these vaccines is not much in
comparison to what is naturally occurring within the body. So, in short,
formaldehyde is naturally inside our cells and in our fluids. When in such
a small amount, our body eliminates it easily and therefore prevents
formaldehyde from accumulating and becoming toxic.

Seems like formaldehyde was a good choice to use over so many other
toxins out there. With a half-life of 1.5 minutes, formaldehyde doesn't

even have the chance to accumulate in the body. So, adding up the formaldehyde in multiple vaccines given over time isn't really an appropriate argument for toxicity. But what if individuals prone to vaccine injuries retain or accumulate formaldehyde?

When the pile gets bigger

We found a study that measured accumulated formaldehyde in the brain. Yes, apparently accumulated formaldehyde *does* exist. The study showed that the more it accumulates, the less there will be "cognitive abilities during human aging"[18]. The more severe the dementia in Alzheimer's disease patients, the higher the formaldehyde accumulation.[19]

Something else the authors of that study observed was when we age, the "accumulation of formaldehyde" prevents "new formation of spatial memory (i.e., learning difficulty)." [20]

Another observation was that in late stage Alzheimer's disease there's "chronic accumulation of hippocampal formaldehyde" which "induces loss of remote memory." What caught our attention was the paper listed a correlation between the presence of both mercury and formaldehyde (as an environmental factor).[21]

This study was not done on children, but on adults with Alzheimer's disease.

We wonder if there's any type of defect in our ability to clear formaldehyde out of the body and that somehow renders the aforementioned short half-life to be irrelevant? Can this formaldehyde accumulation start as early as with the administration of childhood vaccines? Does the combination of formaldehyde and mercury make a difference in children?

Earlier in the chapter, we established that formaldehyde was used to inactivate or kill pathogens and to cross-link cell surface-proteins together. If using our earlier understanding of immune response, is it not possible that our body could create an immune response to formaldehyde?

As a matter of fact, we found a paper describing how alcohol metabolites, which include formaldehyde, have the ability to induce immune response even when an adjuvant (like aluminum) is not used.[22]

As we continued our research, it seemed as if no scientists were sufficiently concerned about formaldehyde in vaccines to study it any further. Unfortunately, most studies have focused on routes other than injections from vaccines. Probably because, compared to their data on non-injected formaldehyde, the minute amounts in vaccines are not considered harmful.

When we looked on websites for the Occupational Safety and Health Administration (OSHA), the Centers for Disease Control and Prevention (CDC) and the National Institute for Occupational Safety and Health (NIOSH), none of them listed injections as a means for formaldehyde exposure.[23][24][25][26]

Seems like the vaccine ingredient motto has become: "It's not a big deal, don't worry about it!"

At the vaccine injection site, even though the formaldehyde is in low concentration, the first thing it will do is latch on to the first available proteins it can get hold of. There should be plenty of proteins right there by the injection site for the formaldehyde molecules to find.

Our immune system is always hard at work. Since the site of entry is a break in the skin, our immune cells (innate immunity) will flock to the site. When our proteins have been altered by formaldehyde, the macrophages don't recognize them as a part of the body anymore. They will attack and gulp them down. From there, the macrophage escorts the formaldehyde to other locations in the body such as our organs, lymph nodes (T cells and B cell hangouts) and the brain.

When formaldehyde enters a cell, it attaches itself to the DNA strand. This can be concerning because it can cause certain genes to be turned off when we need them turned on. Once this happens it's very difficult to reverse or turn back on.[27]

Formaldehyde has been studied and used for a very long time. Even as far back as 1945 we humans were using it in vaccines.

Researcher Dexter French[28], wrote a research paper on using formaldehyde in vaccines.

He expressed concern about its stability:

> *"Formaldehyde, however, owing to the very compact structure of the molecule and its high reactivity, is a particularly versatile reagent with a vast range of possible reactions."*[29]

On the National Institute of Health's (NIH) *Open Chemistry Database*, it says that liquid form of FA (formalin) "is considered a hazardous compound, and its vapor toxic."[30]

It also says:

> *"Formaldehyde is a Standardized Chemical Allergen.*
>
> *"Aqueous formaldehyde is corrosive to carbon steel, [...].*
>
> *"When liquid formaldehyde is warmed to room temp in a sealed ampule, it polymerizes rapidly with the evolution of heat [...]"* [31]

Under the header *Disinfectants*, it defines formaldehyde as:

> *"[...] used on inanimate objects that destroy harmful microorganisms or inhibit their activity. Disinfectants are classed as complete, destroying SPORES as well as vegetative forms of microorganisms, [...]"*[32]

It sounds to us like formaldehyde in liquid form can have harmful effects. We understand the dosing is the argument here, but a *safe dose* is not the same for every single person.

And how does formaldehyde react when combined with all the other toxins in the vaccines?

Synergism

Unfortunately, in vaccines, it seems the synergistic effects of the toxins have never been studied. However, other fields of study have expressed concern for toxic synergism and researched the synergistic effects it has on our bodies when exposed to multiple toxins simultaneously. As with the paper we mentioned earlier regarding accumulation of formaldehyde, this study shows synergistic effects when in contact with mercury. So, for some reason, it appears scientists in other fields test for toxic synergism, just not those who are testing for vaccine safety.

We were able to find a study that focused specifically on synergistic effects, but, of course, it was unrelated to vaccines. It was a Chinese study done to see if co-exposure of air pollutants and formaldehyde could cause Alzheimer's disease (AD). Among the pollutants, which are listed in the paper, was aluminum (Al).[33]

The interesting part of the study was the fact that when the mice were exposed to toxins alone or formaldehyde alone, it "had little or no effect on the mouse brain." When the mice were co-exposed to air pollutants and formaldehyde, it "had a significant synergistic adverse effect."[34]

These adverse effects included "significant cognitive decline." Other observations included deterioration of the blood-brain barrier (BBB) and damages to the hippocampus, which plays an important part of creating memory.[35]

Another observation they made was an abnormally induced expression of tau proteins which:

> *"[...] destroy the stability of microtubules and axonal transport, eventually causing neuronal death, and inducing the occurrence of neurodegenerative diseases."* [36]

The paper also states that "[t]hese safe levels for alone exposure turned into dangerous at co-exposure."[37]

So, there you have it. At least in this study, they show that levels considered safe became highly toxic when combined.

We now have two studies showing synergism. One showing synergism between formaldehyde and mercury, the other showing synergism between formaldehyde and aluminum. With the immune system working overtime on eliminating all these toxins, surely other functions must suffer.

When a developing brain is desperately fighting off the toxins, could this battle possibly be diverting energy and other resources away from other important developmental processes? We're not sure of the answer, but when the body is sick, it will shut down some of its functions in order to give energy to fight the sickness. We are theorizing here that the brain may perhaps react in a similar manner.

Chapter 13: The right amount

[1] Mitkus, R.J., Hess, M.A., and Schwartz S.L. (2013). Pharmacokinetic modeling as an approach to assessing the safety of residual formaldehyde in infant vaccines. *Vaccine*, 31(25), 2738-2743

[2] East Carolina University. (n.d.). *Formalin*. Retrieved from www.ecu.edu/cs-admin/oehs/envmgmnt/Formalin.cfm

[3] Ibid.

[4] Ibid.

[5] Nie, C. L., Wang, X. S., Liu, Y., Perrett, S., & He, R. Q. (2007). Amyloid-like aggregates of neuronal tau induced by formaldehyde promote apoptosis of neuronal cells. *BMC neuroscience*, 8, 9. doi:10.1186/1471-2202-8-9

[6] Chen, K., Maley, J., and Yu, P.H. (2006). Potential implications of endogenous aldehydes in beta-amyloid misfolding, oligomerization and fibrillogenesis. *J Neurochem*, 99(5), 1413–1424.

[7] Hempen, B. (1996). Reduction of acetylated alpha-tubulin immunoreactivity in neurofibrillary tangle-bearing neurons in Alzheimer's disease. *J Neuropathol Exp Neurol*, 55(9), 964-972.

[8] American Cancer Society. (2014, May 23). *Formaldehyde*. Retrieved from www.cancer.org/cancer/cancer-causes/formaldehyde.html

[9] Centers for Disease Control and Prevention. (2018, July 12). *Ingredients of Vaccines - Fact Sheet*. Retrieved from www.cdc.gov/vaccines/vac-gen/additives.htm

[10] Metz, B., Jiskoot, W., Hennink, W.E., Crommelin, D.J., and Kersten, G.F. (2003). Physicochemical and immunochemical techniques predict the quality of diphtheria toxoid vaccines. *Vaccine*, 22(2), 156–167

[11] Dr. Sherri. (2013, January 29). *Formaldehyde in Vaccines*. Retrieved from www.tenpennyimc.com/2013/01/29/formaldehyde-in-vaccines/

[12] Sullivan, J.B. Jr. and Krieger, G.R. (2001) *Clinical Environmental Health and Toxic Exposures* (p. 1008). Philadelphia: Lippinscott Williams & Wilkins.

[13] The units in the research paper are in mmol, and not mg. To convert mmol to mg, we need to know the molecular weight of FA, which is 30.031 g/mol. So, 0.1 mmol/L therefore equals 3.0 mg/L.
www.convertunits.com/from/moles+Formaldehyde/to/grams

[14] Miao, J., Lu, J., Zhang, Z., Tong, Z., and He, R. (2013). The Effect of Formaldehyde on Cell Cycle Is in a Concentration-dependent Manner. *Progress in Biochemistry and Biophysics*, 40(7), 641-651.

[15] Geggel, L. (2016, March 3). *How Much Blood Is in the Human Body?*. Retrieved from www.livescience.com/32213-how-much-blood-is-in-the-human-body.html

[16] Children's Hospital of Philadelphia. (2018, May 14). *Vaccine Ingredients – Formaldehyde*. Retrieved from www.chop.edu/centers-programs/vaccine-education-center/vaccine-ingredients/formaldehyde

[17] Note that polio vaccine is shown in percentage: 0.02 (100µg/.5ml dose).

[18] Tong, Z., Han, C., Qiang, M., Wang, W., Lv, J., Zhang, S., ... He, R. (2015). Age-related formaldehyde interferes with DNA methyltransferase function, causing memory loss in Alzheimer's disease. *Neurobiology of Aging*, 36(1), 100-110.
[19] Ibid.
[20] Ibid.
[21] Ibid.
[22] Thiele, G.M., Tuma, D.J., Willis, M.S., Miller, J.A., McDonald, T.L., Sorrell, M.F., and Klassen, L.W. (1998). Soluble proteins modified with acetaldehyde and malondialdehyde are immunogenic in the absence of adjuvant. *Alcohol Clin Exp Res*. 22(8), 1731-1739.
[23] Agency for Toxic Substances & Disease Registry. (2015, May 12). *Toxic Substances Portal – Formaldehyde*. Retrieved from www.atsdr.cdc.gov/toxfaqs/tf.asp?id=219&tid=39 and Centers for Disease Control and Prevention. (2004, October 6). *Formaldehyde*. Retrieved from www.cdc.gov/niosh/ipcsneng/neng0275.html
[24] Occupational Safety and Health Administration. (n.d.). *OSHA FactSheet*. Retrieved from www.osha.gov/OshDoc/data_General_Facts/formaldehyde-factsheet.pdf
[25] Centers for Disease Control and Prevention. (1994, May). *Formaldehyde*. Retrieved from www.cdc.gov/niosh/idlh/50000.html and United States Environmental Protection Agency. (2000, January). *Formaldehyde*. Retrieved from www.epa.gov/sites/production/files/2016-09/documents/formaldehyde.pdf
[26] United States of America Consumer Product Safety Commission. (2013). *Update on Formaldehyde*. Retrieved from www.cpsc.gov/PageFiles/121919/AN%20UPDATE%20ON%20FORMALDEH YDE%20final%200113.pdf
[27] Woodrow, C.M. (2011). *While Science Sleeps*. United States of America: Amazon.
[28] Iowa State University. (2012, February 3). *Special Collections and University Archives*. Retrieved from www.findingaids.lib.iastate.edu/spcl/arch/rgrp/13-35-12.html
[29] Anson, M.L. and Edsall, J.T. (1945) *Advances in Protein Chemistry* (p. 332). New York: Academic Press Inc.
[30] National Center for Biotechnology Information. PubChem Compound Database (n.d.). *Formaldehyde*. Retrieved from www.pubchem.ncbi.nlm.nih.gov/compound/712 www.pubchem.ncbi.nlm.nih.gov/compound/formaldehyde
[31] National Center for Biotechnology Information. PubChem Compound Database (n.d.). *Formaldehyde*. Retrieved from www.pubchem.ncbi.nlm.nih.gov/compound/712 www.pubchem.ncbi.nlm.nih.gov/compound/formaldehyde#section=Ionization-Potential
[32] National Center for Biotechnology Information. PubChem Compound Database (n.d.). *Formaldehyde*. Retrieved from www.pubchem.ncbi.nlm.nih.gov/compound/712 www.pubchem.ncbi.nlm.nih.gov/compound/formaldehyde#section=Pharmacology

[33] Liu, X., Zhang, Y., Luo, C., Kang, J., Li, J., Wang, K., Ma, P., ... Yang, X. (2017). At seeming safe concentrations, synergistic effects of PM2.5 and formaldehyde co-exposure induces Alzheimer-like changes in mouse brain. *Oncotarget*, 8(58), 98567-98579. doi:10.18632/oncotarget.21637
[34] Ibid.
[35] Ibid.
[36] Ibid.
[37] Ibid.

CHAPTER 14

Polysorbate 80, the ambusher

*"I freed a thousand slaves. I could have freed
a thousand more if only they knew they were
slaves."*

*~**Harriet Tubman** (American abolitionist
and political activist)*

Many ingredients go into the making of a vaccine. Once you've inserted them all into the vaccine batch, you need a way to blend them together. If you have ever spent time in the kitchen cooking or baking, (we'd imagine) you know that there are certain ingredients that don't mix, like oil and water, unless they receive a helping hand.

The same goes for vaccines. In order to blend vaccine ingredients together a change in temperature won't do the trick. A substance that stabilizes or blends the vaccine ingredients together is needed. One such ingredient is polysorbate 80 (p80), often referred to as tween 80. It's a vaccine stabilizer, surfactant or emulsifier, which means something that evenly blends the ingredients together that wouldn't otherwise blend.

When p80 is exposed to oxygen, it automatically forms formaldehyde (FA). In a Swedish study from 1997, it was shown to form the same amount of formaldehyde as found in "allergic individuals." P80 already had allergens in it before being exposed to oxygen. But, after the exposure, new additional allergens were formed. The researchers conclude that it's also a "possibility that allergenic compounds can be formed during storage and handling"[1].

When p80 is added to the vaccine, it becomes aggravated. This was shown in a study from 2002 which comments that:

> *"Literature studies report that the oxidation of polysorbates is greatly accelerated once placed into aqueous solution."*[2]

Oxidation means that the molecule (p80 in this case) is giving away one of its electrons. For instance, when it attaches to an oxygen molecule, it is giving one of its electrons to the oxygen molecule.

A study by the biopharmaceutical company, *Pfizer,* showed the impact formaldehyde and other impurities can have on the proteins used in their pharmaceutical products. The authors of this paper made note of the fact that p80 is efficient at forming formaldehyde:

> *"Both formaldehyde and formic acid can be formed from oxidative degradation of polysorbates."*[3]

The authors don't just concern themselves with polysorbates, of which polysorbate 80 appears most potent, they state that:

> *"These residual impurities and contaminants can potentially impact the protein stability significantly."*[4]

In their conclusion they summarize the limitations of the manufacturing process by saying that:

> *"Although many process-related impurities are routinely monitored, contaminants are generally not, [...]. This is because the level of these contaminants in a drug product is often too low to be detected by traditional analytical methods, and does not lead to serious safety concerns."*[5]

We find their comment that "it does not lead to safety concerns" after stating these "contaminants can potentially impact the protein stability significantly" rather interesting given much of the paper is about safety concerns.

Stormtroopers

Polysorbate 80 has the ability to both form formaldehyde and attack our body.

In previous chapters we talked about how formaldehyde (FA) affects the body. In this chapter we'll explain how p80 attacks the body.

A couple of important concerns we were unable to find papers on was how much of the p80 is converted to formaldehyde once injected and how the increased oxidation affects the process we're about to describe.

The immune process that p80 emulates is called the MAC attack, or in more proper terms, the Membrane Attack Complex (MAC). In order to understand what we mean by that, let's first brush up on what MAC is.

The MAC is a complement cascade that takes place within our innate immune system (first responders). It consists of proteins labeled with the letter "C" and a number (and a letter) that tells you its location in the cascade. A complement basically means that it consists of a bunch of proteins (in the blood) that form a structure (a complex). So, a complement cascade becomes a sort of a domino sequence where each protein activates the next.

There are three different pathways to a MAC. We won't get into any of them in great detail, preferring to refer only to the relevant portion of it for this chapter. The portion that pertains to the p80 in vaccines consists of the proteins C5b through C9. This is called the Terminal Complement Pathway.[6]

When invading substances trigger the immune system, the proteins C5b through C8 link together to form a chain. On the end of this chain, a bunch of C9 proteins form a circle. This chain attempts to attach itself to both our own cells and invader cells. The circle consisting of a bunch of C9s burrow a hole in invading cells, allowing the contents to leak out. This kills the invading cell.

Fortunately, our cells found a way to protect themselves. So, even though the MAC doesn't know the difference between our own cells and invading cells, it leaves our cells alone. This is not only fortunate, but logical in terms of evolution.

On the surface of our cells, we have something called protectin[7]. When this cascade is being assembled and C8 has been added, the protectin steps in and blocks C9 from attaching. This prevents the complement from being completed. Since C9 never gets attached, nothing happens. No drill, no spill.[89]

Unfortunately, there are some germs that have figured this out. They have acquired protectin-like protein on their own cell membrane.[10] HIV, for instance, figured out how to insert this code into its own DNA and therefore blocks the MAC attack.

P80 attacks our cells in a very similar manner to that which our MAC attacks invaders. In addition, the polysorbate 80 also activates C3a, which is an anaphylatoxin, and C5a, which is another anaphylatoxin.[11] Anaphylatoxins trigger all the signs and symptoms of instant anaphylaxis (hypersensitivity). They do this without involving help from antibodies.

The C3a actually causes the B cells (acquired immunity) to respond, while C5a brings in the Th1 cells to strengthen the acquired immune response. This way they're able to recruit immune cells to the site of inflammation, keeping the inflammation fired up.

This makes p80 yet another substance to increase the inflammation process in our body. A question we were unable to find the answer to was whether individuals who have been vaccinated with vaccines containing p80 have a higher incidence of anaphylaxis than individuals vaccinated with vaccines without p80.

P80 has been considered to be a concealed "inductor of anaphylactoid reactions."[1213] What this means is that the protectin on our cell surface that protects us from the MAC attack does not protect us from a p80 attack. When the protectin is not protecting our cells, the cells will be punctured and start leaking. Consequences of this include damaged kidneys, arthritis and nerve damage.[14]

It's in everything

Vitamin E supplements are sometimes given intravenously to babies soon after they are born. Some infants have suddenly died after such a treatment. The authors of a study looking into toxic effects on intravenous administration of vitamin E conclude that:

> *"The life-threatening hazard of such treatment has been attributed mainly to polysorbates that are used as detergents in preparations of vitamin E for intravenous use rather than vitamin E itself."*[15]

Another paper covered p80's role as an ingredient in antiretroviral therapy (ART), which is often used to treat HIV/AIDS patients. Here, the scientists coated nanoparticles with p80 and watched it spread inside the body. They then compared it to a drug not coated with p80.

They found that p80 coated nanoparticles magnified the "delivery into various organs by several fold in comparison to the free drug."[16]

The study also discovered that organs containing numerous macrophages may be the reason for the increased uptake of p80 coated nanoparticles. The macrophages eat the p80 since it is a foreign substance. They will then transfer it straight to our organs, lymph nodes and brain. It was also shown that p80 coated particle "concentration in brain, was seven times higher and in lymph nodes six times higher than that of the free drug."[17]

It appears to be a well-known fact in the medical field that p80 helps drugs across the blood-brain barrier (BBB). One of the papers we looked at concludes:

> "A non specific permeabilization of the BBB, probably related to the toxicity of the carrier, may account for the CNS [Central Nervous System] penetration of [...] and polysorbate 80."[18]

When the permeability of the blood-brain barrier is not being picky or specific about what it's allowing into the brain, our nerve cells become vulnerable to foreign attacks. Continuing on with the paper, the authors also observed that in addition to causing a leaky blood-brain barrier, p80 also caused:

> "[P]otent and prolonged analgesia, [...]. Locomotor activity dramatically decreased in mice [...] also caused occasional mortality."[19]

P80 has also been shown to be toxic to the liver.[20][21] The tricky part with p80 is that it takes very little of it to alter our cells. It changes some of the parts on the cell surface and also some of the functions inside the cell. The tricky part is that it does all this without changing the normal function of the cell.[22]

Perhaps P80 doesn't alter the cell's normal functions, as this study states. That doesn't mean it will not damage or make the cell weaker so other substances have an easier access into our cells.

Another paper on how polysorbate coated particles affects the Central Nervous System (CNS), shows similar results. The authors observed that certain cells in the brain picked up 20 times more of the p80 coated particles than uncoated ones.[23]

The brain has fluid filled cavities called choroid plexuses. These cavities are lined with cells called ependymal (*covering* in Greek) cells, which produce cerebrospinal fluid (CSF).

There is also a sensitive membrane that covers the brain and spinal cord called pia mater (Latin for *tender mother*).

Polysorbate 80 is capable of increasing the space between the ependymal cells. When this happens, unwanted substances are able to squeeze through between the cells and make the brain and spinal cord toxic.[24]

Safety Data Sheet

Unfortunately, all the research papers we found on p80 were unrelated to vaccines. As with the other substances, in order to truly understand the potential effects when these are injected into the body, we dug deeper to gain a better understanding of p80. One of these angles in this case was looking at the Safety Data Sheet (SDS) for p80.

We discovered that safety data sheets often lack crucial information. Even so, we hoped to find information as it relates to being injected, as in liquid form in a vaccine. What we found was not exactly what we hoped for:

> *"May cause adverse reproductive effects based on animal test data. No human data found. May cause cancer based on animal test data. No human data found. May affect genetic material (mutagenic)"*[25].

We wondered what the potential chronic health effects were:

> *"CARCINOGENIC EFFECTS: Not available.*
> *MUTAGENIC EFFECTS: Not available.*
> *TERATOGENIC EFFECTS: Not available.*
> *DEVELOPMENTAL TOXICITY: Not available.*
> *Repeated or prolonged exposure is not known to aggravate medical condition… Exposure Limits: Not available."*[26]

According to this safety data sheet (SDS), the *Routes of Entry: Inhalation. Ingestion* does not include injection. Nowhere does it mention this substance (p80) should be injected.

This substance is injected into, dare we say, the entire human population, yet the SDS fails to cover this route of entry. When a route is this commonly used, it should at least warrant a mention in the safety data sheet.

The SDS continues:

> *"Special Remarks on Chronic Effects on Humans: May cause adverse reproductive effects based on animal test data. No human data found. May cause cancer based on animal test data. No human data found. May affect genetic material (mutagenic)"*[27]

What about other effects that are not chronic? Have these effects been tested on humans?

The toxic effect segment states:

> *"Ingestion: This material is not likely to cause irritation upon ingestion. [...] Animal studies have shown it to cause cardiac changes, changes in behavior (altered sleep time) and weight loss (upon repeated or prolonged ingestion). However, no similar human data has been reported."*[28]

Here the SDS says it's not likely to cause irritation. It appears to us this statement is based on the fact that there haven't been any reports on it. But if it's causing harm in animal studies, shouldn't that be grounds for observational studies in humans? Why is there no human data? It's very surprising to us that when a substance is tested on animals, and the observations are cause for concern, the very product is approved for use in humans.

Nor do we understand how a product with such concerning results from animal testing is not at least included in observational studies in humans, since it's already being injected in us.

It feels like such a substance, until proven safe, should come with a warning label made known to the user. If we understand correctly, it's not safe for human studies, but it is safe to use in humans without properly testing it first. How does that work?

We took a look at p80 SDS sheet from another company just to compare. We looked at the section covering *chronic effects, mutagenicity, carcinogenicity, reproductive toxicity, specific target organ toxicity, specific organ toxicity,* and there was only one entry:

> *"No information available."*[29]

When there is little or no data available, how can the National Fire Protection Association (NFPA) show in the diamond (health hazard information label) that health hazard is only at 1, meaning it is *slightly hazardous?*[30]

Neither of these SDS sheets include injection as a potential point of entry. The toxicology fact sheet on p80 on the website for National Institutes of Health (NIH) doesn't say that p80 may be injected into the body.[31]

If it's being injected into practically every single person, shouldn't that qualify for at least a single mention on the SDS sheet?

We would assume the manufacturer is aware that one of the routes of entry being used is via injection. It's surprising to us, then, that they aren't required to either list it as one of the options, or warn against using it in injections. We don't see how the safety hazard of 1 (meaning it is slightly hazardous) can apply to vaccines.

One of our concerns after reading the SDS sheets is whether the demonstrated toxic effects of p80 in animals, including damage to the uterus and ovaries leading to infertility, applies to humans as well.

Chapter 14: Polysorbate 80, the ambusher

[1] Bergh, M., Magnusson, K., Nilsson, J.L, and Karlberg, A.T. (1997). Contact allergenic activity of Tween 80 before and after air exposure. *Contact Dermatitis*, 37(1), 9-18.

[2] Maggio, E.T. (2012). Polysorbates, peroxides, protein aggregation, and immunogenicity– a growing concern. *J. Excipients and Food Chem*, 3(2).

[3] Wang, W., Ignatius, A.A., and Thakkar, S.V. (2014). Impact of Residual Impurities and Contaminants on Protein Stability. *J Pharm Sci*, 103(5), 1315-1330.

[4] Ibid.

[5] Ibid.

[6] Svar Life Science AB (formerly Euro Diagnostica). (n.d.). *Lytic part of the complement pathway*. Retrieved from www.complementsystem.se/terminal-pathway

[7] Also referred to as CD59, but we prefer calling it protectin, because it describes what it is for. It is a protector of the cell. Any name that ends with -in is a protein. So the word means a protein that protects.

[8] Nesorgikar, P., Spiller, B., and Chavez, R. (2012). The complement system: History, pathways, cascade and inhibitors. *Eur J Microbiol Immunol (Bp)*, 2(2), 103-111.

[9] Meri, S., Morgan, B. P., Davies, A., Daniels, R. H., Olavesen, M. G., Waldmann, H., & Lachmann, P. J. (1990). Human protectin (CD59), an 18,000-20,000 MW complement lysis restricting factor, inhibits C5b-8 catalysed insertion of C9 into lipid bilayers. *Immunology*, 71(1), 1-9.

[10] Roitt, I.M, and Delves, P.J., (Eds.). (1998). *Encyclopedia of Immunology*. U.S.: Academic Press.

[11] Weiszhar, Z., Czúcz, J., Révész, C., Rosivall, L., Szebeni, J., and Rozsnyay, Z. (2012). Complement activation by polyethoxylated pharmaceutical surfactants: Cremophor-EL, Tween-80 and Tween-20. *Eur J Pharm Sci*, 45, 492-498.

[12] Coors, E.A., Seybold, H., Merk, H.F., and Mahler, V. (2005). Polysorbate 80 in medical products and nonimmunologic anaphylactoid reactions. *Ann Allergy Asthma Immunol*, 95(6), 593-599.

[13] Price, K.S. and Hamilton, R.G. (2007). Anaphylactoid reactions in two patients after omalizumab administration after successful long-term therapy. *Allergy Asthma Proc*, 28(3), 313-319.

[14] National Center for Biotechnology Information, U.S. Nation. (n.d.). *Search results*. Retrieved from www.ncbi.nlm.nih.gov/pubmed?cmd=retrieve&list_uids=17635812,16951374,16859686,16494864,15457473

[15] Pacifici, M.G. (2016). Effects of Vitamin E in Neonates and Young Infants. *Int J Pediatr*, 4(5), 1745-1757.

[16] Jenita, J.L., Chocalingam, V., and Wilson, B. (2014). Albumin Nanoparticles Coated with Polysorbate 80 as a Novel Drug Carrier for the Delivery of Antiretroviral drug—Efavirenz. *Int J Pharm Investig*, 4(3), 142–148.

[17] Ibid.

[18] Olivier, J.C., Fenart, L., Chauvet, R., Pariat, C., Cecchelli, R., and Couet, W. (1999). Indirect evidence that drug brain targeting using polysorbate 80-coated polybutylcyanoacrylate nanoparticles is related to toxicity. *Pharm Res*, 16(12), 1836-1842.

[19] Ibid.

[20] Giannattasio, F., Salvio, A., Varriale, M., Picciotto, F.P., Di Costanzo, G.G., and Visconti, M. (2002). Three cases of severe acute hepatitis after parenteral administration of amiodarone: the active ingredient is not the only agent responsible for hepatotoxicity. *Ann Ital Med Int*, 17(3): 180-184.

[21] Ellis, A.G., Crinis, N.A., and Webster, L.K. (1996). Inhibition of etoposide elimination in the isolated perfused rat liver by Cremophor EL and Tween 80. *Cancer Chemother Pharmacol*, 38(1), 81-87.

[22] Hirama, S., Tatsuishi, T., Iwase, K., Nakao, H., Umebayashi, C., Nishizaki, Y., ... Oyama, Y. (2004). Flow-cytometric analysis on adverse effects of polysorbate 80 in rat thymocytes. *Toxicology*, 199(2-3), 137-143.

[23] Ramge, P., et al. "Polysorbate-80 coating enhances uptake of polybutylcyanoacrylate (PBCA)-nanoparticles by human and bovine primary brain capillary endothelial cells." *Eur J Neurosci*. 2000, 12(6):1931-1940.

[24] Olivier, J.C., Unger, R.E., Oltrogge, J.B., Zenker, D., Begley, D., Kreuter, J., and Von Briesen, H. (1999). Indirect evidence that drug brain targeting using polysorbate 80-coated polybutylcyanoacrylate nanoparticles is related to toxicity. *Pharm Res*, 16(12), 1836-1842.

[25] Chemicals & Laboratory Equipment. (2013, May 21). *Medical Safety Data Sheet for Polysorbate 80*. Retrieved from www.sciencelab.com/msds.php?msdsId=9926645

[26] Ibid.

[27] Ibid.

[28] Ibid.

[29] Bronson and Jacobs. (2018, February 21). *Polysorbate 80*. Retrieved from www.msds.orica.com/pdf/shess-en-cds-010-000000031369.pdf

[30] Chemicals & Laboratory Equipment. (2013, May 21). *Medical Safety Data Sheet for Polysorbate 80*. Retrieved from www.sciencelab.com/msds.php?msdsId=9926645

[31] U.S. National Library of Medicine. (2010, October 15). *Polysorbate 80*. Retrieved from www.toxnet.nlm.nih.gov/cgi-bin/sis/search2/r?dbs+hsdb:@term+@rn+9005-65-6

CHAPTER 15

Toxins—Accumulative harmful effects

*"The truth is, natural organisms have
managed to do everything we want to do without
guzzling fossil fuels, polluting the planet or
mortgaging the future."*

~Janine Benyus *(American writer).*

In a research paper from 1993, the researchers injected neonatal female rats with polysorbate 80 (p80). The effect was "accelerated maturation" which led to ovaries "without corpora lutea." These are a cluster of cells that form inside the ovary early on in the pregnancy. They produce progesterone, and "degenerative follicles." The follicles are a sac inside the ovary that carries the oocyte (egg).[1]

So, we have known this for at least 25 years, yet when it's added to vaccines scientists don't bother to test it. It appears that once these substances have been added to the vaccine, the concern for toxicity magically disappears.

P80 attaches very well to Aluminum (Al). Now you have an adjuvant, like aluminum, coating the vaccine-antigen together with p80, and other substances within the vaccine. This new larger vaccine-antigen is then escorted across the blood-brain barrier (BBB). Note that anything that can cross the blood-brain barrier can most likely cross the gut-brain barrier. When in contact with p80, the blood-brain barrier has been shown to become weakened and penetrated, resulting in complications ranging from seizures to death.[23]

In 2005 a study was published on "organic compounds leached from uncoated rubber stoppers in prefilled syringes containing polysorbate 80"[4]. After looking at patient data from 2001 to 2003, the researchers conclude:

> *"[...] leachates from uncoated rubber syringe stoppers caused the increased incidence of PRCA"*[5].

Pure red cell aplasia (PRCA) is the type of anemia where the bone marrow stops producing red blood cells. So, the question is how much p80 does it take to cause harm? Obviously, it depends on the individual. But we doubt very much that the amount of p80 contained in the rubber stopper which contaminated the prefilled syringe, was more than barely a trace amount. And yet it was shown to have serious effects.

The transformer

Polymyxin b, an antibiotic used in vaccines, has been shown to work in toxic synergy with p80. This means the toxic effect of both substances is potentiated.

This was known at least as far back as 1971, when it was noted in a study on the synergism between the two substances. It was observed that polymyxin b and p80 worked together to cause "leakage, death and lysis" to bacterial cells. The explanation was that p80 changes the surface membrane of the bacterial cell. This allows polymyxin b a better access to the cell.[6]

Not much is said about this substance in regards to vaccinations, so we had to be a little more creative in our research. We wanted to see what happens to the p80 substance itself once inside our body. It turns out our body tries to break it apart into individual molecules.

P80 consists mainly of oleic acid, ethylene oxide (EtO) and sorbitol. It has about 20 moles of EtO for every mole of sorbitol.[7]

We wondered if these molecules could be harmful to us after p80 was broken apart as the sweet-smelling gas EtO[8] is considered quite hazardous. The International Programme on Chemical Safety (IPCS) wrote about EtO in their Chemical Safety Information from Intergovernmental Organizations (INCHEM). They mentioned studies from various US states and countries, such as Sweden and Italy, where cancers of all sorts had been related to EtO exposure.[9]

The International Agency for Research on Cancer (IARC) reviewed the potency of EtO and observed that in mammalian cells, its:

> *"[...] effects include gene mutations, micronucleus formation, chromosomal aberrations, cell transformation, unscheduled DNA synthesis, sister chromatid exchange, and DNA strand breaks."*[10]

Sounds to us like the perfect recipe for causing cancer. And on that note, how much does vaccine research take into account long term, harmful health effects as opposed to merely childhood health risks? For example, how much research takes into account whether vaccines in childhood could cause autoimmune disorders in early adulthood, or cancer in middle-age, or Alzheimer's disease (AD) in old age?

IARC has EtO listed as having *'limited evidence* in humans for breast cancer and Leukemia/lymphoma.[11] On IARCs website, EtO is classified as group 1 agent[12], which means it is a *"Carcinogenic to humans"*[13]

According to the Agency for Toxic Substances & Disease Registry, EtO is incompatible with, among other things, aluminum[14]. This means it will react harshly when combined.

Although EtO is not directly injected into the body, it's still a biproduct of an injected substance. The fact that it's not meant to be injected into the body is patently evident given none of the safety and exposure information to be found on this element includes injection.

The CDC also mentions EtO on their website:

> *"Ethylene oxide [...] resulting in cellular and tissue dysfunction and destruction. Evidence for human exposure to this chemical is the presence of ethylene oxide adducts of DNA and hemoglobin. Direct contact with liquid ethylene oxide or solutions."*[15]

Another factor that makes it so difficult to assess research on chemicals or substances in relation to vaccines is that injecting infants, toddlers, older children or adults are not necessarily comparable with each other.

Although not vaccine-related, the CDC's website confirms this when they state that:

> *"Children do not always respond to chemicals in the same way that adults do."*[16]

Something to keep in mind is that it can take up to three days to experience symptoms because it can take this long for nerve and respiratory reactions to present themselves.[17] This may be a reason why symptoms often are not considered to be related to vaccines.

During vaccine safety testing, the observational period often doesn't last long enough to record delayed reactions. Yet, those are the studies on which vaccine safety is based.

A study was performed on pregnant women in South Africa who were exposed to EtO when sterilizing medical equipment. It was found that there seemed to be a strong connection between EtO exposure and "spontaneous abortion [...] and pregnancy loss [...]"[18].

According to the Environmental Protection Agency (EPA):

> *"Many countries have banned the use of ETO on spices and other food due to concerns for public exposure to ETO and its reaction products. [...] due to its classification as a known human carcinogen and genotoxic agent. [...] some of the countries that have banned the use of ETO on spices (and other foods) include: Belize, China, the European Union (EU, currently numbering 25 countries), Australia, and Japan."[19]*

As we can see, there's research out there showing the serious effects these substances may have on our cells. The dilemma is not whether these substances are toxic, but whether the amount used in vaccines, or the biproducts once injected, is enough to cause concern. Keeping in mind EtO isn't directly in the vaccine but presents itself after our body has dissected p80.

Polysorbate 80 reacts to yet another vaccine substance. Namely mercury. Mercury was removed from almost all vaccines, but is still found in some multi-dose vials to prevent bacterial contamination. An example of such vaccine is the influenza vaccine[20]. Even though mercury was removed from childhood vaccines, there are still residual amounts left over from the manufacturing process.

A study we came across revealed that p80 is very efficient at removing mercury from contaminated water.[21] This sounds good right? Read on…

If p80 is attracting mercury, we can only assume it is likely some of the mercury is being escorted to the brain. So, if we receive traces of mercury in the vaccines or are exposed to mercury from other sources, and receive a p80 containing vaccine, then a mercury-free vaccine could still potentially cause mercury accumulation in the brain.

Chapter 15: Toxins – Accumulative harmful effects

[1] Gajdová, M., Jakubovsky, J. and Války, J. (1993). Delayed effects of neonatal exposure to Tween 80 on female reproductive organs in rats. *Food Chem Toxicol,* 31(3), 183-190.

[2] Dib, B. and Falchi, M. (1996). Convulsions and death induced in rats by Tween 80 are prevented by capsaicin. *Int J Tissue React,* 18(1), 27-31.

[3] Azmin, M.N., Stuart, J.F. and Florence, A.T. (1985). The distribution and elimination of methotrexate in mouse blood and brain after concurrent administration of polysorbate 80. *Cancer Chemother Pharmacol,* 14(3), 238-242.

[4] Boven, K., Stryker, S., Knight, J., Thomas, A., van Regenmortel, M., Kemeny, D.M., ... Casadevall, N. (2005). The increased incidence of pure red cell aplasia with an Eprex formulation in uncoated rubber stopper syringes. *Kidney Int,* 67(6), 2346-2353.

[5] Ibid.

[6] Brown, M.R.W. and Winsley, B.E. (1971). Synergism between Polymyxin and Polysorbate 80 against *Pseudomonas aeruginosa. Journal of General Microbiology,* 68: 367-373

[7] The United States Pharmacopeial Convention. (2017, August 1). *Polysorbate 80.* Retrieved from www.usp.org/sites/default/files/usp/document/harmonization/excipients/polys orbate_80.pdf

[8] U.S. National Library of Medicine. (2009, April 18). *Ethylene Oxide.* Retrieved from www.toxnet.nlm.nih.gov/cgi-bin/sis/search2/r?dbs+hsdb:@term+@rn+75-21-8

[9] Liteplo, R.G. and Meek, M.E., Health Canada, Ottawa, Canada., and Lewis, M., Environment Canada, Ottawa, Canada. (2003). *Ethylene Oxide.* Retrieved from www.inchem.org/documents/cicads/cicads/cicad54.htm#9.2

[10] Ibid.

[11] International Agency for Research on Cancer. (2018, November 2). *List of Classifications by cancer sites with sufficient or limited evidence in humans, Volumes 1 to 123.* Retrieved from www.monographs.iarc.fr/wp-content/uploads/2018/07/Table4.pdf

[12] International Agency for Research on Cancer. (n.d.). *List of classifications, Volumes 1–123.* Retrieved from www.monographs.iarc.fr/ENG/Classification/latest_classif.php

[13] International Agency for Research on Cancer. (2018, November 9). *Agents Classified by the IARC Monographs, Volumes 1–123.* Retrieved from www.monographs.iarc.fr/ENG/Classification/index.php

[14] www.atsdr.cdc.gov/mmg/mmg.asp?id=730&tid=133

[15] Ibid.

[16] Ibid.

[17] Ibid.

[18] Gresie-Brusin, D.F., et al. "Occupational exposure to ethylene oxide during pregnancy and association with adverse reproductive outcomes." *Int Arch Occup Environ Health.* 200, 80(7): 559-565. PMID: 17165063. DOI: 10.1007/s00420-006-0163-y

[19] US Environmental Protection Agency Office of Pesticide Programs. Reregistration Eligibility Decision for Ethylene Oxide. March 31, 2008. www.archive.epa.gov/pesticides/reregistration/web/pdf/ethylene-oxide-red.pdf

[20] Agency for Toxic Substances and Disease Registry. (2014, October 21). *Toxic Substances Portal - Ethylene Oxide.* Retrieved from www.fda.gov/BiologicsBloodVaccines/SafetyAvailability/VaccineSafety/UCM096228

[21] Chen, H. R., Chen, C. C., Reddy, A. S., Chen, C. Y., Li, W. R., Tseng, M. J., Liu, H. T., Pan, W., Maity, J. P., … Atla, S. B. (2011). Removal of mercury by foam fractionation using surfactin, a biosurfactant. *International journal of molecular sciences*, 12(11), 8245-8258.

CHAPTER 16

Mercury, the swift traveler

"It does indeed seem absurd that an organic disposition should make beings more fragile, more susceptible to poisons, for in most cases everything in living beings seems disposed to assure them a greater power of resistance."

~**Dr. Charles Richet** *(French physiologist)*

The body has an amazing capacity to take care of itself. It contains highly intricate molecules that work hard at keeping our bodies as healthy as possible. One of the body's very own molecules to do this is glutathione (GSH). Its job is to clean house. It makes sure your cells are not hoarding all kinds of garbage it doesn't need. As diligent as this little molecule is, it is also sensitive to certain toxic exposures. Unfortunately, vaccines are adding hard-to-dodge obstacles in their path.

In order to understand the overall importance of what the glutathione does and the consequences of the potential exposure of some vaccines, we need to first take a look at its function within the body and then see what happens when it's under attack.

Our body is constantly producing glutathione protein molecules. Its superpower is its sticky and stinky sulfur content. Because it is so sticky, heavy metals and toxins, such as free radicals and mercury, stick to it. When materials stick to the glutathione, it takes it out with the *trash* and the unwanted materials end up in our feces. It's not surprising that glutathione also plays a vital role "in normal intestinal function."[1]

Normally, our body just recycles our glutathione, which in turn recycles antioxidants. When our body experiences oxidative stress or is bombarded with too many toxins, it has a hard time keeping up. When this happens, the glutathione is overworked and the body is unable to recycle it fast enough and it gets used up (no more sticky stuff). This means we are no longer recycling our antioxidants to fight off free radicals. This in turn causes oxidative stress. Our battle is taking its toll and cellular functions suffer.

Glutathione (GSH) is extremely important if we want our immune system to work properly.

A paper published in 2014 on glutathione states:

> "GSH also has crucial functions in the brain as an antioxidant, neuromodulator, neurotransmitter, and enabler of neuron survival."[2]

Glutathione is produced in the liquid portion (cytosol) inside our cells. There are many cellular functions that need glutathione in order to operate properly. For instance, glutathione is also in the nucleus where it helps produce and repair DNA. The mitochondria also contain glutathione, the mitochondrial glutathione (mGSH). In this mitochondrial form, it helps keep the cell alive.[3]

Fighting the free radicals

The mitochondria are the parts inside the cells that consume the most oxygen. They contain a lot of antioxidants and detoxifying agents. The most important agent is perhaps the mitochondrial glutathione because it protects the mitochondria from things like premature cell death.[4] The mitochondria are constantly exposed to free radicals, and glutathione is at the forefront fighting against them.

When a cell dies, so does its glutathione content. So, when a cell prematurely dies, the body is losing its glutathione supply.

One of the organs that has the most glutathione is the liver. The kidney is another one with a lot of glutathione. It would therefore not be surprising if a disease of an organ, like the liver, would be related to lack of glutathione in liver cells.

Nor is it surprising that doctors warn that acetaminophen is hard on the liver when you understand that acetaminophen depletes the glutathione (GSH) in the liver cells. It reduces the mitochondrial glutathione (mGSH), which makes the cell more defenseless against free radicals or oxidative stress.[5]

We did some reading on neurological disorders and it seemed many are contributed to oxidative stress and mitochondrial dysfunction.

Scientists say:

> *"[…], a reduction in both cellular and mitochondrial GSH levels results in increased oxidative stress and a decrease in mitochondrial function […]."*[6]

One cannot help but wonder about the vaccines' role in all this. As our brain uses a lot of oxygen, it is prone to much oxidative stress. Compared to a healthy active person, the brain of an infant or an elderly person is less likely to be able to fight the stress. This can lead to such things as Alzheimer's disease (AD) and Parkinson's disease in the elderly.[7]

We wonder then if it is possible it could lead to neurological disorders, such as autism spectrum disorder (ASD) in children.

Toxin magnet

The liver is an important organ that delivers glutathione into the blood and to other organs.[8] When it comes to protecting our organs, the glutathione's most important job is to detoxify. It's therefore also important to have plenty of glutathione in our lungs. As you know, lungs are a major oxygen-containing organ and can also be full of toxins from the air we breathe.

One toxin presented to us in some vaccines is thimerosal, even though mostly in only trace amounts. Glutathione draws it out of the body via the kidney and liver. Once thimerosal is in liquid, it decomposes into ethylmercury hydroxide and ethylmercury chloride.[9] Glutathione helps eliminate the ethylmercury. If our glutathione system doesn't function properly, it won't be able to help get rid of the ethylmercury.[10]

Glutathione is one of our main defenders against the toxic effects thimerosal has on our cells. When our cells are attacked by toxic levels of thimerosal, it depletes the glutathione within our cells.[11]

After our main defenders, glutathione, have been depleted and we continue to be repeatedly exposed to thimerosal, it's not so surprising that our cells are easily invaded and killed. Perhaps lack of glutathione can be a genetic defect in some individuals? If such a thing exists, could some children suffer extreme reactions when vaccinated, even with just trace amounts of toxins?

As a matter of fact, after looking it up, glutathione deficiency exists. An example is glutathione synthetase deficiency. Individuals with this disorder are unable to produce glutathione. This specific disorder comes in a mild, moderate or severe form.

Those with the severe form may experience:

> "[...] seizures; a generalized slowing down of physical reactions, movements, and speech (psychomotor retardation); intellectual disability; and a loss of coordination (ataxia). Some people [...] develop recurrent bacterial infections."[12]

We feel it's safe to assume that those who have some type of glutathione deficiency may react severely to vaccines. In addition, we find the above descriptions similar to that of severe reactions to vaccines. Perhaps vaccines can affect glutathione production even in healthy babies and consequently cause the above symptoms.

Girls and boys

Another link in the chain is uncovered in some of the research into neuroblastoma cell lines. Neuroblastoma cells are cancer cells often used when researching nerve cells. Neuroblasts are immature or naïve nerve cells that haven't been told yet what they are.

Several online articles mention that boys are more prone to adverse reactions to thimerosal than girls. How can this be? Thimerosal affects the neuroblastoma cells by telling it to self-destruct. That sounds like a good thing, don't we want cancer cells to self-destruct? As great as that sounds, it's not so great considering the fact it will do it to normal cells as well. How can this be gender-based?

One reason males may be more prone to adverse reactions to thimerosal is the relationship between testosterone and nerve cell development. Testosterone causes almost an instantaneous increase in calcium (Ca) inside the neuroblastoma cells. The calcium is extremely important in growing neurons for proper brain function and proper function of the nervous system.

Researchers injected neuroblastoma cells with a small amount of thimerosal to see what would happen to the nerve cell. They saw physical changes in the cells, including changes in the cell surface, the membrane. The researchers watched as the cell withered away. They also noticed that important substances were leaking out of the mitochondria and identified these substances as ones that play an active role in cell destruction. Therefore, these events caused the cell to self-destruct prematurely.[13]

When the cells are exposed to too much testosterone it causes damage which may change a person's behavior. Suicidal thoughts being one such change. We found a paper that explains the effects testosterone has on nerve cells. The authors of the paper showed a correlation between overstimulation of this self-destruction process and disorders such as Alzheimer's disease and Huntington disease.[14]

Sounds familiar? The effect of ethylmercury on neuroblastoma cells is quite similar to that of over-active testosterone levels in neuroblastoma cells. Not only is it similar to testosterone, but it also mimics formaldehyde's (FA) effect on the microtubular structure in the cytoskeleton.[15] So not only is it messing with the self-destruction code, but the mercury also tears down our microtubules as we talked about in the book's section on formaldehyde.

A healthy production of testosterone is necessary in order to keep the calcium in check inside the cell. Too much testosterone, can kill nerve cells. The above research paper concludes that "effects of testosterone on neurons will have long term effects on brain function."[16] Mercury affects the production of testosterone.[17][18]

The study tested this by using estrogen as well. Estrogen did not have any effect on the cell's integrity. Their explanation was "that normal levels of testosterone are necessary" in order to have the right amount of calcium "to maintain homeostasis"[19].

When we have an increased level of testosterone, this changes the calcium signal and results in the killing of nerve cells.[20] It has also been shown that estrogen is able to keep the calcium (Ca) levels stable. This maintains the functional homeostasis and protects mitochondria from oxidative stress.[21]

The next question is why estrogen doesn't do the same damage. The paper continues by explaining how estrogen is able "to protect neurons from a number of toxic insults"[22]. Not only that, but we learned it also protected the cell from dying by being exposed to heavy metals such as mercury. Estrogen has also been shown to protect us from diseases such as Alzheimer's disease (AD) and Parkinson's.[23] It's also known to protect the nerves by ensuring the mitochondria are functioning properly.

The disturbance of testosterone and estrogen production in a developing body can potentially seriously affect the neurons. With mercury playing a role in this disturbance, especially in testosterone production, why are we concerned about its effect in terms of childhood vaccines? Mercury was removed from childhood vaccines and the trace amounts we spoke of earlier doesn't seem to be enough to elicit a concern of this magnitude.

In order to understand how this can potentially cause serious issues in children who have some kind of immune weakness, we need to look at what mercury-free (trace amount) vaccines means to a compromised immune system.

Chapter 16: Mercury, the swift traveler

[1] Lushchak, V.I. (2012). Glutathione Homeostasis and Functions: Potential Targets for Medical Interventions. *Journal of Amino Acids*, 2012: 736837. www.dx.doi.org/10.1155/2012/736837

[2] Morris, G., Anderson, G., Dean, O., Berk, M., Galecki, P., Martin-Subero, M., and Maes, M. (2014). The Glutathione System: A New Drug Target in Neuroimmune Disorder. *Mol Neurobiol*, 50(3), 1059–1084

[3] Lushchak, V.I. (2012). Glutathione Homeostasis and Functions: Potential Targets for Medical Interventions. *Journal of Amino Acids*, 2012: 736837.

[4] Marí, M., Morales, A., Colell, A., García-Ruiz, C., & Fernández-Checa, J. C. (2009). Mitochondrial glutathione, a key survival antioxidant. *Antioxidants & redox signaling*, 11(11), 2685-2700.

[5] Vendemiale, G., Grattagliano ,I., Altomare, E., Turturro, N. and, Guerrieri, F. (1996). Effect of acetaminophen administration on hepatic glutathione compartmentation and mitochondrial energy metabolism in the rat. *Biochem Pharmacol*, 52(8), 1147-1154.

[6] Marí, M., Morales, A., Colell, A., García-Ruiz, C., & Fernández-Checa, J. C. (2009). Mitochondrial glutathione, a key survival antioxidant. *Antioxidants & redox signaling*, 11(11), 2685-2700.

[7] Schultz, J.B., Lindenau, J., Seyfried, J., and Dichgans, J. (2000). Glutathione, oxidative stress and neurodegeneration. *Eur J Biochem*, 267(16), 4904-4911.

[8] Song, Z., Cawthon, D., Beers, K., and Bottje, W.G. (2000). Hepatic and extra-hepatic stimulation of glutathione release into plasma by norepinephrine in vivo. *Poult Sci*, 79(11), 1632-1639.

[9] Geier, D.A., King, P.G., Hooker, B.S., Dórea, J.G., Kern, J.K., Sykes, L.K., and Geier, M.R. (2015). Thimerosal: Clinical, epidemiologic and biochemical studies. *Clinica Chimica Acta*, 444, 212-220.

[10] Westphal, G.A., Schnuch, A., Schulz, T.G., Reich, K., Aberer, W., Brasch, J., ... Hallier, E. (2000). Homozygous gene deletions of the glutathione S-transferases M1 and T1 are associated with thimerosal sensitization. *Int Arch Occup Environ Health*, 73(6), 384-388.

[11] James, S.J, Slikker, W. 3rd., Melnyk, S., New, E., Pogribna, M., and Jernigan, S. (2005). Thimerosal neurotoxicity is associated with glutathione depletion: protection with glutathione precursors. *Neurotoxicology*, 26(1), 1-8.

[12] NIH.U.S. (2018, December 18). National Library of Medicine. Glutathione synthetase deficiency. Retrieved from www.ghr.nlm.nih.gov/condition/glutathione-synthetase-deficiency

[13] Humphrey, M.L., Cole, M.P., Pendergrass, J.C., and Kiningham, K.K. (2005). Mitochondrial mediated thimerosal-induced apoptosis in a human neuroblastoma cell line (SK-NSH). *Neurotoxicology*, 26(3), 407-416.

[14] Estrada, M., Varshney, A., and Ehrlich, B. (2006). Elevated Testosterone Induces Apoptosis in Neuronal Cells. *J Biol Chem*, 281(35), 25492-25501

[15] University of Calgary. [steffyweffy777]. (2007, May 15). *How Mercury Causes Brain Neuron Damage – Uni. of Calgary.* [Video file]. Retrieved from www.youtube.com/watch?v=XU8nSn5Ezd8

[16] Estrada, M., Varshney, A., and Ehrlich, B. (2006). Elevated Testosterone Induces Apoptosis in Neuronal Cells. *The Journal of Biological Chemistry*, 281(35), 25492-25501

[17] Heath, J.C, Abdelmageed, Y., Braden, T.D., and Goya, H.O. (2012). The Effects of Chronic Ingestion of Mercuric Chloride on Fertility and Testosterone Levels in Male Sprague Dawley Rats. *Journal of Biomedicine and Biotechnology*, 2012, 815186

[18] Chen, H., Pechenino, A. S., Liu, J., Beattie, M. C., Brown, T. R., & Zirkin, B. R. (2008). Effect of glutathione depletion on Leydig cell steroidogenesis in young and old brown Norway rats. *Endocrinology*, 149(5), 2612-2619.

[19] Estrada, M., Varshney, A., and Ehrlich, B. (2006). Elevated Testosterone Induces Apoptosis in Neuronal Cells. *J Biol Chem*, 281(35), 25492-25501

[20] Ibid.

[21] Simpkins, J. W., Perez, E., Wang, X., Yang, S., Wen, Y., & Singh, M. (2009). The potential for estrogens in preventing Alzheimer's disease and vascular dementia. *Therapeutic advances in neurological disorders*, 2(1), 31-49.

[22] Ibid.

[23] Olivieri, G., Novakovic, M., Savaskan, E., Meier, F., Baysang, G., Brockhaus, M., and Müller-Spahn, F. (2002). The effects of beta-estradiol on SHSY5Y neuroblastoma cells during heavy metal induced oxidative stress, neurotoxicity and beta-amyloid secretion. *Neuroscience*, 113(4), 849-855.

CHAPTER 17

Mercury, the ungodly element

*"[E]ating a peppermint before bed justifies
not brushing your teeth because it gives the same
flavour"*

~Unknown.

Now that we know a little bit more about what's going on inside our cells when we are exposed to heavy metals, let's to take closer look at mercury. According to the United States Environmental Protection Agency (EPA), there are three forms of mercury:

> *"[...] elemental mercury, inorganic mercury compounds (primarily mercuric chloride), and organic mercury compounds (primarily methyl mercury). All forms of mercury are quite toxic, and each form exhibits different health effects."*[1]

Thimerosal is a type of organic mercurial compound.[2] Mercury (Hg) is elemental and a heavy liquid state. Methyl Mercury (CH_3Hg) is organic and a solid state and Thimerosal ($C_9H_9HgNaO_2S$) is organic and a solid state.

As you can see, these are three different compounds.[3] Both methylmercury and thimerosal are organic and solid. Note that it's in the form of thimerosal and not ethylmercury. As mentioned earlier, thimerosal turns into ethylmercury when in liquid.

When reading the vaccine ingredient label, take notice whether it says thimerosal or mercury. Thimerosal contains about 50% mercury. So, when it says the thimerosal in a vaccine is "50 micrograms per 0.5 mL dose"[4], which is a normal size dose[5] for injection, that means that it contains about "25 micrograms of mercury per 0.5 mL dose."[6]

You've most likely heard that mercury has been removed from vaccines. So it was, at least for the most part. Thimerosal, which is the ethylmercury component used in vaccines, is found in vaccines for influenza, tetanus, Japanese encephalitis, meningococcal and Td.[7]

There used to be a lot more mercury in vaccines and it was added for a very good reason. During the vaccine manufacturing process, it is likely the vaccine vial becomes contaminated with living organisms. It's also likely that when performing multiple needle pokes into a multi-dose vial, it becomes contaminated with living organisms.

Mercury was added to multidose vials in order to protect us from being injected with these unknown living organisms. According to the FDA, the amount of thimerosal in vaccines "kills the specified challenge organisms and is able to prevent the growth of the challenge fungi."[8]

The FDA gives a quick history of how thimerosal has been used in vaccines since the 1930s, stating:

> *"Since then, thimerosal has a long record of safe and effective use preventing bacterial and fungal contamination of vaccines, with no ill effect established other than minor local reactions at the site of injection."*[9]

How much is trace?

In the CDC's pink book (referenced above), it says there can be up to 0.3 µg of mercury left in the vaccine after thimerosal has been removed. It's important to note there is a difference between thimerosal and mercury. We have noticed when discussing mercury in vaccines with others, they use thimerosal and mercury interchangeably as if they were the same thing.

The FDA states:

> *"Since 2001, all vaccines manufactured for the U.S. market and routinely recommended for children ≤ 6 years of age have contained no thimerosal or only trace amounts (≤ 1 microgram of mercury per dose remaining from the manufacturing process), with the exception of inactivated influenza vaccine."*[10]

We noticed the CDC and the FDA show two different cut-offs for what constitutes trace amounts. The CDC specifies 0.3 μg in one dose:

> *"Evaluated detection limits were 0.3 μg TM [thimerosal] and 3.0 μg Al, which corresponds to the smallest, but possible to recognize, visible peak."*[11]

The FDA doesn't appear to agree with this lower limit, because as stated above, they specify 1.0 μg per dose as an accepted amount in their thimerosal-free vaccines.

We thought it strange that these two organizations would have such variation in what defines a *trace amount*. We looked into it a little closer and found the discrepancy to be even larger than expected. The CDC is actually referring to thimerosal, while the FDA is referring to mercury.

As mentioned above, the 0.3 μg thimerosal is derived from the fact that it's the *limit of detection* for the methods used to test for thimerosal.[12] This means if there is 0.29 μg thimerosal in the vaccine, it will show up as no thimerosal detected. According to the FDA, these vaccines are labeled "thimerosal-free"[13]. The CDC demonstrated slightly more concern, and in 2001, they:

> *"[R]efused even to express a preference for thimerosal-free vaccines, despite the fact that thimerosal had been removed from almost every childhood vaccine produced for use in the United States."*[14]

When it comes to what the FDA considers a trace amount (1 μg mercury or less/dose) amounts to 2 μg thimerosal or less/dose.

So, when the FDA states there's either no thimerosal or trace amounts of thimerosal in the vaccines, they are in reality saying thimerosal is anywhere from 0 μg to 2 μg.

According to the FDA website, in 1999 the FDA conducted an in-depth analysis on thimerosal and its use in childhood vaccines. They "found no evidence of harm from the use of thimerosal as a vaccine preservative, other than local hypersensitivity reactions."[15]

What is interesting here is that the FDA doesn't seem to be concerned that thimerosal causes *local hypersensitive reactions*. This is interesting because, taking local hypersensitivity into account, the Pittman-Moore Company found Merthiolate (aka thimerosal) to be:

"[...] unsatisfactory as a preservative for serum intended for use on dogs"[16]

So, Merthiolate is not desirable for uses in dogs, but in humans it's okay?

Let's get back to the trace amounts and work on those numbers a little to see what they mean. One vaccine dose is 0.5 ml. We are going with the CDC's guidelines where the maximum trace amount of mercury allowed is 0.3 µg/0.5 ml. This is the same as 600 parts per billion (ppb). [17]

The United States Environmental Protection Agency's (EPA) safety levels are calculated in mg/l and ppb. According to the EPA, the maximum amount of inorganic mercury allowed in drinking water is 0.002 mg/l or 2 ppb. This means the max trace amounts in vaccines is 300 times above the maximum allowed in drinking water.[18] By the way, *inorganic* is considered less harmful than *organic* mercury.

Note that we are comparing inorganic mercury (drinking water) to thimerosal, which is organic mercury. This is why we mentioned the different types of mercury in the beginning of this chapter. We want you to be aware that although it's all mercury, it's not all the same.

We also want to mention that by the time mercury reaches the brain, it has changed into an inorganic form. When ethylmercury is transported out of the muscle and into the tissues, it quickly converts into an inorganic form of mercury. This has to do with the red blood cells' ability to convert it.[19]

A multidose influenza vaccine contains 25 µg of thimerosal. As mentioned above, 1.0 µg/l is the same as 1 ppb. Since there is 25 µg in 0.5 ml dose, this is the same as 50,000 ppb in one single flu shot.

According to the Healthcare Environmental Resource Center, a waste substance that "contains more than 0.2 mg per liter mercury, the waste is considered hazardous."[20] A quick reminder, 0.2 mg per liter mercury is the same as 200 ppb mercury. Thimerosal contains 50% mercury.

According to our calculations, this means that a substance needs to contain 400 ppb of thimerosal to be considered hazardous waste. Compared to the 50,000 ppb thimerosal in the influenza vaccine, we can safely say that it contains more than a hundred times more thimerosal than the legal limit of a toxic waste.

Chapter 17: Mercury, the ungodly element

[1] United States Environmental Protection Agency. (2000, January). *Mercury Compounds*. Retrieved from www.epa.gov/sites/production/files/2016-09/documents/mercury-compounds.pdf

[2] The Centers for Disease Control and Prevention (CDC). (2009, November). *Mercury*. Retrieved from www.cdc.gov/biomonitoring/pdf/Mercury_FactSheet.pdf

[3] Broussard, L.A., Hammett-Stabler, C.A., Winecker, R.E., and Ropero-Miller, J.D. (2002). The Toxicology of Mercury. *laboratorymedicine*, 8(33), 614-625.

[4] U.S. Food and Drug Administration. (2018, February 2). *Thimerosal and Vaccines*. Retrieve from www.fda.gov/biologicsbloodvaccines/safetyavailability/vaccinesafety/ucm096228

[5] Immunization Action Coalition. (2018, October). *Administering Vaccines: Dose, Route, Site, and Needle Size*. Retrieved from www.immunize.org/catg.d/p3085.pdf

[6] U.S. Food and Drug Administration. (2018, February 2). *Thimerosal and Vaccines*. Retrieve from www.fda.gov/biologicsbloodvaccines/safetyavailability/vaccinesafety/ucm096228

[7] The Centers for Disease Control and Prevention (CDC). (2015, April). *Pink Book-Appendix B-Vaccines*. Retrieved from www.cdc.gov/vaccines/pubs/pinkbook/downloads/appendices/appdx-full-b.pdf

[8] U.S. Food and Drug Administration. (2018, February 5). *Thimerosal in Vaccines Questions and Answers*. Retrieved from www.fda.gov/biologicsbloodvaccines/vaccines/questionsaboutvaccines/ucm070430.htm

[9] U.S. Food and Drug Administration. (2018, February 5). *Thimerosal in Vaccines Questions and Answers*. Retrieved from www.fda.gov/biologicsbloodvaccines/vaccines/questionsaboutvaccines/ucm070430.htm

[10] U.S. Food and Drug Administration. (2018, February 5). *Thimerosal in Vaccines Questions and Answers*. Retrieved from www.fda.gov/biologicsbloodvaccines/vaccines/questionsaboutvaccines/ucm070430.htm

[11] Zareba, M., Sanecki, P.T, and Rawski, R. (2016). Simultaneous Determination of Thimerosal and Aluminum in Vaccines and Pharmaceuticals with the Use of HPLC Method. *Acta Chromatographica*, 28(3), 299–311.

[12] Ibid.

[13] U.S. Food and Drug Administration. (2018, February 5). *Thimerosal in Vaccines Questions and Answers*. Retrieved from www.fda.gov/biologicsbloodvaccines/vaccines/questionsaboutvaccines/ucm070430.htm

[14] Burton, D. (2003, May30). *Mercury in Medicine*. [Congressional Report]. Retrieved from www.gpo.gov/fdsys/pkg/CREC-2003-05-21/html/CREC-2003-05-21-pt1-PgE1011-3.htm

[15] U.S. Food and Drug Administration. (2018, February 5). *Thimerosal in Vaccines Questions and Answers*. Retrieved from www.fda.gov/biologicsbloodvaccines/vaccines/questionsaboutvaccines/ucm070430.htm

[16] Burton, D. (2003, May30). *Mercury in Medicine.* [Congressional Report]. Retrieved from www.gpo.gov/fdsys/pkg/CREC-2003-05-21/html/CREC-2003-05-21-pt1-PgE1011-3.htm

[17] endmemo. (n.d.). *Microgram/ml ↔ Part per billion Conversion.* Retrieved from www.endmemo.com/sconvert/ug_mlppb.php

[18] United States Environmental Protection Agency. (2018, March 22). *National Primary Drinking Water Regulations.* Retrieved from www.epa.gov/ground-water-and-drinking-water/national-primary-drinking-water-regulations

[19] Carneiro, M.F., Oliveira Souza, J.M., Grotto, D., Batista, B.L., de Oliveira Souza, V.C., and Barbosa, F. Jr. (2014). A systematic study of the disposition and metabolism of mercury species in mice after exposure to low levels of thimerosal (ethylmercury). *Environmental Research*, 134, 218-227.

[20] Healthcare Environmental Resource Center. (n.d.). *Mercury in Healthcare Facilities.* Retrieved from www.hercenter.org/hazmat/mercury.cfm

CHAPTER 18

Mercury, it's everywhere

"Man was born free, and he is everywhere in chains."

~Jean-Jacques Rousseau (French philosopher).

Although not a part of the childhood vaccine schedule, the influenza vaccine is still given to children and childbearing women. We wonder what kind of impact this can have on a developing fetus or a breastfeeding infant. Even if what authorities say about mercury in the vaccine being safe or not toxic enough on its own is true, how does it fare when in contact with other vaccine ingredients?

It appears that our bodies have become a toxic dumping ground, but it's okay, because only trace amounts are being dumped each time, right?

It's important to note not all flu vaccines contain thimerosal. There are flu vaccines available that are labeled "thimerosal-free." We encourage those who decide to be vaccinated against the flu to ask which flu vaccine you're about to receive.

The ethylmercury in vaccines has often been compared to the toxic methylmercury contaminating our waters and the fish we eat. Because of this, pregnant women, for instance, are told not to consume fish. Many argue that we are injecting infants and pregnant mothers with a substance they are advised not to eat.

In one article Paul Offit says:

> *"Ethylmercury is broken down and excreted much more rapidly than methylmercury. Therefore, ethylmercury (the type of mercury in the influenza vaccine) is much less*

likely than methylmercury (the type of mercury in the environment) to accumulate in the body and cause harm."[1]

This very article was reviewed by Dr. Paul Offit himself in 2018. It's not our intent to pick on Dr. Offit. We are merely using him as a source due to his respected standing within the vaccine field in the scientific community. We feel confident his statements are based on what is considered to be solid opinions within the scope of vaccine research.

A 2002 paper by Pichichero, which supports Dr. Offit's statement, is often used as a reference to prove mercury in vaccines is safe. This paper "aimed to measure concentrations of mercury in blood, urine, and stools of infants who received such vaccines."[2] Interestingly, the authors stated that "allergic reactions have been rarely noted, but no harmful effects have been reported."[3] They linked this statement to a paper from 1988. How about in the 14 years since the study? Were there no reports of value in those years? I'm sure any one of you can find reports of this sort.

After collecting samples from both test group and control group, the researchers found that "[m]ercury was undetectable in most of the urine samples from the infants in this study."[4]

A test group consists of subjects receiving a substance being tested. In this case it's mercury. A control group consists of subjects *not* receiving the substance being tested. These groups are then compared to each other to observe any impact the substance may have.

In the stool samples from infants in the test group, the researchers did find mercury, mostly inorganic mercury. This isn't surprising given we now know thimerosal turns into inorganic mercury. And after finding out MSG eliminates mercury through the stool, this is to be expected. If you have been exposed to mercury then it should be there (in the stool) just as you'd see in healthy individuals exposed to mercury. The concern would be if there was no mercury measured in the stool.

Stool samples from infants in the control group were not collected.

How can the researchers compare the importance of finding mercury in the stool of the mercury-exposed test group? To us, the logical answer would be that it is an indicator the mercury is being excreted, but we'd like to see the amount excreted being compared to the amount of mercury being injected.

We're not sure how relevant their findings are because, as we understand it, all they are saying is that it appears the GSH is clearing out the mercury as it's supposed to do or that the body is actively eliminating the toxin. These are healthy infants, so this is to be expected. But the paper makes no mention of the expected amount of mercury to be excreted when injected with the vaccines these infants were given. Nor does it say anything about the elimination of mercury of infants with weakened immune response.

Since they didn't collect stool sample from the control group, in order to compare and to see if dietary sources contaminated with mercury could be a factor, they chose nine other babies (unrelated to the study) who had not been injected with thimerosal-containing vaccine. The babies in this group, which was less than half the size of the regular control group, turned out to have a "significantly lower" amount of mercury in their stool. This is only to be expected and not at all surprising.

God only knows why they deviated from the study design in this manner, omitting the control group infants and picking nine other infants who were not a part of the study, is a mystery to us. They didn't explain this.

The researchers also measured the blood half-life of ethylmercury by measuring the mercury blood levels consistently over many days. In the end they estimated the half-life to be seven days. This means that when the mercury was no longer measurable in the blood, it was assumed to be cleared out of the body.

Even though the researchers measured mercury levels in the infants, no blood samples were collected in the first 72 hours.

Could there be reasons, other than excretion, for mercury to leave the bloodstream? How about traveling to the brain with help of, for instance, polysorbate 80? Could this not explain the lack of mercury in the blood? We feel concerns of this caliber should warrant a proper study comparing levels of excreted mercury to injected mercury.

If not all sources are being measured, it's difficult to accept a definitive conclusion.

Three years later, in 2005, another study was published comparing methylmercury to thimerosal in vaccines. This study was performed on macaque monkeys and focused on the mercury levels in the brain, not the urine or the stool.

The study was designed to see if the mercury dose in the vaccine was safe since it was based on methylmercury rather than ethylmercury.

The researchers state that:

> *"Studies in preterm infants indicate that blood levels of Hg after just one vaccination (hepatitis B) increase by >10-fold to levels above the US EPA guidelines."*[5]

The macaque monkeys in both the ethylmercury group and the methylmercury group showed similar levels of mercury immediately after distribution.

The methylmercury seemed to have a much higher tendency to accumulate in the blood while the ethylmercury cleared out very quickly from the blood. Instead of being eliminated from the body, the scientists noticed it was escaping across the blood-brain barrier (BBB).

When kidneys were tested, much higher levels of mercury were found in the thimerosal-injected group. This would correlate with the fact that mercury sticks to GSH and our kidneys have a large amount of GSH.

When measuring mercury levels in the brain, it was noted ethylmercury left much higher levels of inorganic mercury than did methylmercury ("up to 71% vs. 10%").

While ethylmercury is quick to leave the blood and enter our organs, including the brain, we can't see how this makes it safer than methylmercury which stays in the blood longer before it's cleared out.

Life of mercury

What about the half-life of organic vs. inorganic mercury? "The estimated half-life of organic Hg in the brain" is about 37 days and "The estimated half-life of inorganic Hg in the brain [...] varied greatly across some regions of the brain, from 227 days to 540 days."[6]

The researchers continue stating that:

> *"In other regions, the concentrations of inorganic Hg remained the same (thalamus) or doubled (pituitary) 6 months after exposure to MeHg had ended"*[7].

Their finding appears to be that the ethylmercury clears the blood quicker, but isn't being eliminated from the body, rather it's traveling to the brain and other organs, including the kidneys, while methylmercury lingers in the blood longer before it reaches the brain.

Therefore:

> *"Consequently, MeHg is not a suitable reference for risk assessment from exposure to thimerosal-derived Hg."[8]*

Another study concludes "that MeHg does not appear to be a good model for EtHg-containing compounds."[9] Yet, the official guidelines don't seem to make this distinction.

Drs. *Thomas Verstraeten* and *Frank DeStefano*, performed a study assessing "the possible toxicity of thimerosal-containing vaccines (TCVs) among infants."[10]

They conclude:

> *"No consistent significant associations were found between TCVs and neurodevelopmental outcomes."[11]*

Regarding the lifespan of ethylmercury from vaccine in the blood, a research summary from the Health & Human Services Committee, states:

> *"The half life is 5–7 days, meaning that half the injected dose of mercury leaves the blood in that time period, on average. There is considerable individual variation. [...] exposures from non-vaccine sources would increase the blood mercury levels."[12]*

Through other research, we know that even though the mercury has left the bloodstream, it doesn't mean it has left the body. The message is a little confusing. The researchers say the half-life is 5–7 days, but that's when it is being measured in the blood. But what if in 5–7 days the ethylmercury has vanished because it has traveled to the brain and not because of its half-life? Maybe this is not the true half-life for mercury in blood, but rather a measure of how long it takes until it travels to organs.

We decided to look into this so we visited our favorite webpage on chemicals, the National Institutes of Health's (NIH) open chemistry database. We found what we were looking for in *section 8.7 Biological Half-Life*.[13] The NIH linked their source to the Drugbank.[14] The NIH, or the Drugbank, had completely different estimates for the half-lives of thimerosal. They link their sources to a research paper in the *Environmental Journal*[15] and the University of Minnesota[16]. Unfortunately, during the final polishing of this book, the latter source doesn't appear to be available any longer.

The NIH summarizes its sources to:

> "*Estimated half-lives (in days) were 8.8 for blood, 10.7 for brain, 7.8 for heart, 7.7 for liver and 45.2 for kidney [L1685]. The long half-life of ethylmercury (~50 days on average in humans) results in accumulation that may be harmful to the developing fetal brain, as it is more susceptible to organomercurial compounds than the adult brain [L1687].*"[17]

That being said, in section 8.5 they refer to Pichichero's study, which we mentioned at the start of this chapter.

It states that:

> "*Estimated blood half-life of ethylmercury was 7 days.*"[18]

Their discussion doesn't end here. In section 8.8 they continue by explaining that thimerosal's behavior is not well understood. For those who understand chemistry, you may prefer to read the section for clarification. However, for the rest of us, it says, in a nutshell, that thimerosal has the ability to release calcium from our cells. This results in an excess amount of calcium outside the cell. Because our body uses calcium for various functions, this transfer of calcium can mess up those functions.

Since ethylmercury is a lipophilic cation, meaning it is positively charged and dissolves in fat, it can cross the blood-brain barrier.

This is an important note, because, as this section states:

> "*It has been demonstrated that lipophilic cations accumulate inside mitochondria [...].*[19]

After reviewing various sources, it has now become apparent to us that research papers on the life of mercury in our body can reach various conclusions depending on which source is used to interpret the data.

We feel confident in the validity of our concern that ethylmercury, or thimerosal, travels to the brain and our other organs rather than being completely excreted from the body.

Skulls & bones

Thimerosal has two Globally Harmonized Systems (GHS) hazard statements. One is from the European Chemicals Agency (ECHA) and the other from NITE-CMC. The ECHA statements are a collection of statements from 84 companies. Let's see what these agencies think about thimerosal.

ECHA has labeled thimerosal with health hazard and environment hazard warnings inclusive of the universal skull & crossbones images. That agency informs us thimerosal is both toxic and fatal when swallowed, fatal if it comes in contact with your skin or is inhaled. When there is an extended contact with thimerosal, it can damage the organs.[20]

NITE-CMC have labeled thimerosal similarly along with it being toxic if swallowed. They don't mention it's deadly, as ECHA did. Instead of saying it's fatal at skin contact, they say that it "[m]ay cause an allergic reaction." What they do mention, which ECHA doesn't, is the fact that there's a chance it can cause genetic defects and cancers. Both agencies agree on the damage it causes organs.[21]

The SDS sheet for thimerosal classifies it as class 6.1, which means it is poisonous.[22] What does it say the *Potential Acute Health Effects* are?

> *"Hazardous in case of skin contact (irritant), of ingestion, of inhalation. Slightly hazardous in case of eye contact (irritant). Severe over-exposure can result in death."*[23]

What about *Potential Chronic Health Effects?*

> *"CARCINOGENIC EFFECTS: Not available. MUTAGENIC EFFECTS: Mutagenic for mammalian somatic cells. TERATOGENIC EFFECTS: Not available. DEVELOPMENTAL TOXICITY: Not available. The substance may be toxic to kidneys, liver, spleen, bone marrow, central nervous system (CNS)."*[24]

The *Special Remarks* on the toxic effects on humans are too long to list. They seem to cover just about any adverse health effect known to Man, and they detail such a wide variety of signs and symptoms.

The SDS sheet also states that thimerosal reacts adversely to oxidizing agents. These take electrons away from other molecules. As you may remember, polysorbate 80 (p80) has an electron to give away. Oxygen is an oxidizing agent[25], so it takes the electron that p80 is giving away.

Our red blood cells carry oxygen on their surface. Thimerosal reacts badly to oxygen. When thimerosal enters blood, it's converted from organic form into inorganic form.

We're not chemists and find it difficult to connect the dots with all the research data we've gathered. Nevertheless, we feel there is more dot-connecting to be done in this area.

A study was performed using *micro- and nanomolar concentrations* of thimerosal to mimic the amounts used in products such as vaccines. After incubating thimerosal in live cell cultures for six hours, it became toxic. The researchers observed that even in these miniscule amounts, the thimerosal "rapidly induce membrane and DNA damage and initiate [...] apoptosis in human neurons and fibroblasts."[26]

Apoptosis means cell death. It's confusing to us to understand how this is even a discussion. We understand that most infants are healthy and *appear to be* vaccinated without any harm. But are they really? What about when symptoms present themselves months or years down the road?

More children are developing allergies than ever before. More children are developing learning difficulties than ever before. More children are developing gut issues than ever before. More children are developing neural disorders than ever before.

There could be many other immune system weaknesses that our children develop, which we are unaware of.

Society has gone through major changes in the past century with vaccines being but one of those changes. Despite that, it's a change that impacts children all over the world, regardless of living conditions, nutrition, race, color or creed.

Chapter 18: Mercury, it's everywhere

[1] The Children's Hospital of Philadelphia. (2018, April 24). *Vaccine Ingredients – Thimerosal.* Retrieved from www.chop.edu/centers-programs/vaccine-education-center/vaccine-ingredients/thimerosal

[2] Pichichero, M.E., Cernichiari, E., Lopreiato, J., and Treanor, J. (2002). Mercury concentrations and metabolism in infants receiving vaccines containing thiomersal: a descriptive study. *The Lancet*, 360(9347), 1737–1741.

[3] Ibid.

[4] Ibid.

[5] Burbacher, T. M., Shen, D. D., Liberato, N., Grant, K. S., Cernichiari, E., & Clarkson, T. (2005). Comparison of blood and brain mercury levels in infant monkeys exposed to methylmercury or vaccines containing thimerosal. *Environmental health perspectives*, 113(8), 1015-1021.

[6] Ibid.

[7] Ibid.

[8] Ibid.

[9] Harry, G.J., Harris, M.W., and Burka, L.T. (2004). Mercury concentrations in brain and kidney following ethylmercury, methylmercury and Thimerosal administration to neonatal mice. *Toxicol Lett*, 154(3), 183-189.

[10] Verstraeten, T., Davis, R.L., DeStefano, F., Lieu. T,A,, Rhodes. P,H,, Black. S,B.. ... Vaccine Safety Datalink Team. (2003). Safety of thimerosal-containing vaccines: a two-phased study of computerized health maintenance organization databases. *Pediatrics*, 112(5), 1039-1048.

[11] Ibid.

[12] Aposhian, H.V., Debold, V., El-Dahr, J.M.S., Herbert, M.R., Hornig, M., James, S.J., ... Walker, S. (2006, February 22). *Summary of Science on Thimerosal Effects at Vaccine-Relevant Doses.*[Research summary]. Retrieved from www.autismbo.startlogic.com/pdf/ScienceSummary.pdf

[13] National Center for Biotechnology Information, U.S. National Library of Medicine. (2018, December 15). *Metabolism/Metabolites.* Retrieved from www.pubchem.ncbi.nlm.nih.gov/compound/thimerosal#section=Metabolism-Metabolites

[14] Drugbank. (2018, December 16). *General References.* Retrieved from www.drugbank.ca/drugs/DB11590#reference-L1685

[15] Carneiro, M.F., Oliveira Souza, J.M., Grotto, D., Batista, B.L., de Oliveira Souza, V.C., and Barbosa, F. Jr. (2014). A systematic study of the disposition and metabolism of mercury species in mice after exposure to low levels of thimerosal (ethylmercury). *Environmental Research*, 2014, 134, 218-227.

[16] www.enhs.umn.edu/current/5103_spring2003/mercury/mercdose.html

[17] National Center for Biotechnology Information, U.S. National Library of Medicine. (2018, December 15). *Metabolism/Metabolites.* Retrieved from www.pubchem.ncbi.nlm.nih.gov/compound/thimerosal#section=Metabolism-Metabolites

[18] National Center for Biotechnology Information, U.S. National Library of Medicine. (2018, December 15). *Absorption, Distribution and Excretion*. Retrieved from www.pubchem.ncbi.nlm.nih.gov/compound/thimerosal#section=Absorption-Distribution-and-Excretion

[19] National Center for Biotechnology Information, U.S. National Library of Medicine. (2018, December 15). Biological Half-Life. Retrieved from www.pubchem.ncbi.nlm.nih.gov/compound/thimerosal#section=Biological-Half-Life

[20] National Center for Biotechnology Information, U.S. National Library of Medicine. (n.d.). *Thimerosal*. Retrieved from www.pubchem.ncbi.nlm.nih.gov/compound/thimerosal#section=GHS-Classification&fullscreen=true

[21] Ibid.

[22] United States Department of Transportation. (2018, October 16). *How to Comply with Federal Hazardous Materials Regulations*. Retrieved from www.fmcsa.dot.gov/regulations/hazardous-materials/how-comply-federal-hazardous-materials-regulations

[23] Science Lab.com Chemicals & Laboratory Equipment. (2013, May 21). *Material Safety Data Sheet Thimerosal MSDS*. Retrieved from www.sciencelab.com/msds.php?msdsId=9925236

[24] Ibid.

[25] Wikipedia. (2018, December 16). *Oxidizing agent*. Retrieved from httpswww.en.wikipedia.org/wiki/Oxidizing_agent

[26] Baskin, D.S., Ngo, H., and Didenko, V.V. (2003). Thimerosal induces DNA breaks, caspase-3 activation, membrane damage, and cell death in cultured human neurons and fibroblasts. *Toxicol Sci*, (2), 361-368.

CHAPTER 19

Monosodium glutamate—Fire away!

"The human brain has 100 billion neurons, each neuron connected to 10 thousand other neurons. Sitting on your shoulders is the most complicated object in the known universe."

~*Michio Kaku* *(American theoretical physicist)*

Vaccines need to be shipped from the manufacturing laboratory to their many destinations such as medical clinics and hospitals. In order to ensure they remain stable during shipping and storage, a substance to help vaccines maintain their integrity is added to their list of ingredients. One such additive is Monosodium glutamate (MSG).

Like many other vaccine ingredients MSG has been shown to affect our body, especially our nerves. Glutamate is not just a vaccine ingredient, it's also an excitatory amino acid present in the human brain. This means it causes excitement. If its function is messed with in any way, it can become toxic to our nerves.[1]

In order to understand how this happens, we have to understand how a nerve cell works. The easiest way for us to do this is to look at the nerve cell as having four parts: dendrites, a body, axon and axon terminals.

Inside the nerve cell body, you'll find the mitochondria, DNA and other organelles. The dendrites is where you receive electrical impulses. These impulses are coming from the axon terminals of another nerve cell. They go from axon terminal and over to the dendrites. The cells never actually touch, instead the impulses rely on the action potential in bringing the message across to the axon terminals. This is how a message can be shot across to another nerve cell. [2][3]

Action potential is the rise and fall of movement along the axon. Reminiscent of a yoyo-like movement.[4] The action potential shoots the message across the axon by recharging the message with a new action potential at each *Node of Ranvier,* which are the gaps between the myelin sheaths along the axon. When a nerve cell doesn't have the protection of a myelin sheath, the message takes a lot longer to process as it needs constant action potentials to move forward, rather than just at the *Nodes of Ranvier.* We have attached a YouTube video that shows an animation of this[5].

Saying we have a lot of synapses wouldn't really explain the vastness of our network. Maybe this quote will put it into perspective:

> *"In the cerebral cortex alone, there are roughly 125 trillion synapses, which is about how many stars fill 1,500 Milky Way galaxies."*[6]

To recap what we just explained, after a dendrite has received electrical impulses from axon terminal of a neighboring nerve cell, they travel down the axon. We need to ensure the message gets across fast and smooth. This is done by covering the axon with myelin sheath, which kind of looks like a row of bricks with a small gap between each brick. These gaps are called the *Nodes of Ranvier* and are filled with sodium (Na) and potassium (K). This is where action potentials are recharged. You can say they are kind of like charging stations.

The electrical impulses slide safely under the protection of the myelin sheath and each time they hit a *Node of Ranvier,* they become recharged and shot forward. In other words, this creates the energy needed to launch the message across the myelin sheath and over to the next Node of Ranvier for recharge (Saltatory conduction).[7] This makes the message go faster, because it only needs to be reloaded at the *Node of Ranvier,* rather than constantly.

When the myelin sheath is damaged, because of how much slower the signal is being transferred, it becomes much like a bad Internet connection. Like watching a film that is constantly buffering.

At the axon terminals which are at the end of the axon you find multiple vacuoles. Inside these vacuoles are neurotransmitters. They help the electrical impulses to cross over to the dendrite part of the neighboring nerve cell. The most common neurotransmitter in our brain is glutamate. As mentioned, glutamate is an excitatory amino acid. This means it increases the positive charge in the cell and helps shoot the impulse across to the other cell.

On the dendrites on the nerve cells you find glutamate receptors (GluR). There are many different types of GluR and they all have different functions. They are needed for, among other things, proper "learning and memory, motor coordination, pain transmission, and neurodegeneration."[8]

So excited, just can't hide it

As mentioned earlier, glutamate is also excitotoxic. When there is too much glutamate in the space outside the cell, it is "a likely trigger of epileptic seizures"[9]. These seizures can cause a lifelong injury to our nerves.[10] This happens if there's too much glutamate or if it's hypersensitive. Both scenarios lead to over-excitation.

When there's too much excitement going on, it affects the cell's ability to produce energy and it starts producing more oxidants. This is very important when it comes to killing nerve cells.[11] So basically, the glutamate excites them to death. This can lead to neurodegenerative diseases.[12]

One concern regarding the use of monosodium glutamate (MSG) in vaccines is when it is given to pregnant women. The MSG can get through the placenta and into the tissues of the embryo.[13] Being exposed to MSG this early on can cause a continuous production of free radicals in the brain.[14] This can impair important brain functions.[15] In fact, a study was done in mice where they were "treated neonatally with monosodium glutamate (MSG)" and they ended up developing "learning and memory deficits"[16] in the task they were given to perform.

We carry the most amount of glutamate in our body at age two. From then on it tapers off. During this time, when the glutamate is decreasing, there's not as much need for the glutamate receptors (GluR), so they start adjusting to other tasks.[17] During brain development period, the brain has more GluR than it will have later in life. This means that while we are young, our brain is more vulnerable to nerve cell damage.

This is not a big deal

Dr. Paul Offit does not appear to be concerned about MSG in vaccines having a negative effect on us. In response to spacing out vaccines, he says in his book *Deadly Choices:*

> *"[...] it's the dose that makes the poison — and that spacing out vaccines to avoid exposure to quantities of chemicals so small that they have no chance of causing harm will accomplish nothing."*[18]

His statement was supported in a report which reviewed the "available literature from last 25 years about different clinical trials"[19] performed on both animals and humans by using multiple scientific databases. The authors of the paper bring up various concerns and make no intention of refuting the adverse effects.

They also state a few advantages of consuming MSG. One advantage being "it is used as a fuel for digestive system to enhance body metabolism."[20]

The only time the paper mentions injected glutamate is during a mouse study, but other than that, there's no mention of it. So, in their conclusion, the authors speak of MSG as a food additive, not a vaccine additive.

Like Dr. Offit, they also say:

> *"Excess of everything was bad, so MSG utilization up to a certain level does not have any adverse effects because glutamate is a nutritionally indispensable amino acid."*[21]

Yet again, the various research papers on a substance used in vaccines render different results. When looking at how each substance affects the body, and then combining all the substances and their effects into one big picture, it's clear that our body's immune system is surrounded by invaders coming at it from all directions.

A strong and healthy immune system may have an army of defenders large enough to keep toxins at bay. What about those who have weaknesses, or even a single weakness, in their immune system? While the immune cells are busy fighting, they may not have enough immune cells or strength to cover any other weakness in the body's defense.

Chapter 19: Monosodium glutamate – Fire away!

[1] Institute of Medicine (US) Forum on Neuroscience and Nervous System Disorders. Glutamate-Related Biomarkers in Drug Development for Disorders of the Nervous System: Workshop Summary. Washington (DC): *National Academies Press* (US); 2011. 2, Overview of the Glutamatergic System. Available from: www.ncbi.nlm.nih.gov/books/NBK62187/

[2] Alila Medical Media. [Mark Cervantes]. (2017, June 20). *Action Potential in Neurons, Animation – PHYSIO.* Retrieved from www.youtube.com/watch?v=wkubHJCLDnE

[3] Harvard Extension School. (2018, March 26). *Action Potential in the Neuron.* Retrieved from www.youtube.com/watch?v=oa6rvUJlg7o

[4] Adam. (2011, November 19). *How the action potentials are propagated.* Retrieved from www.youtube.com/watch?v=Sa1wM750Rvs

[5] JCCCvideo (2009, June 25). *The Schwann Cell and Action Potential.* Retrieved from www.youtube.com/watch?v=DJe3_3XsBOg

[6] Moore, E.A. (2010, November 17). *Human brain has more switches than all computers on Earth.*

[7] Wikipedia. (2018, November 4). *Saltatory conduction.* Retrieved from www.en.wikipedia.org/wiki/Saltatory_conduction

[8] Blaylock, R.L. and Strunecka, A. (2009). Immune-Glutamatergic Dysfunction as a Central Mechanism of the Autism Spectrum Disorders. *Curr Med Chem*, 16(2), 157-170.

[9] Eid, T., Thomas, M.J., Spencer, D.D., Rundén-Pran, E., Lai, J.C., Malthankar, G.V., ... de Lanerolle, N.C. (2004).Loss of glutamine synthetase in the human epileptogenic hippocampus: possible mechanism for raised extracellular glutamate in mesial temporal lobe epilepsy. *The Lancet*, 363(9402), 28-37.

[10] Barker-Haliski, M. and White, H.S. (2015). Glutamatergic Mechanisms Associated with Seizures and Epilepsy. *Cold Spring Harbor Perspectives in Medicine*, 015, 5(8): a022863.

[11] Abramov, A.Y., Scorziello, A., and Duchen, M.R. (2007). Three Distinct Mechanisms Generate Oxygen Free Radicals in Neurons and Contribute to Cell Death during Anoxia and Reoxygenation. *Journal of Neuroscience*, 27(5) 1129-1138.

[12] Martinez-Contreras, A., Huerta, M., Lopez-Perez, S., García-Estrada, J., Luquín, S., and Beas Zárate, C. (2002). Astrocytic and microglia cells reactivity induced by neonatal administration of glutamate in cerebral cortex of the adult rats. *J Neurosci Res*, 67(2): 200-210.

[13] Yu, T., Zhao, Y., Shi, W., Ma, R., and Yu, L. (1997). Effects of maternal oral administration of monosodium glutamate at a late stage of pregnancy on developing mouse fetal brain. *Brain Res*, 747(2), 195-206.

[14] Bawari, M., Babu, G.N., Ali, M.M., and Misra, U.K. (1995). Effect of neonatal monosodium glutamate on lipid peroxidation in adult rat brain. *NeuroReport*, 6(4), 650-652.

[15] Kubo, T., Ryutaro, K., Tadao, O., and Koichi, I. (1993). Neonatal glutamate can destroy the hippocampal CA1 structure and impair discrimination learning in rats." *Brain Research*, 616(1–2), 311-314.

[16] Wong, P.T., Neo, L.H., Teo, W.L., Feng, H., Xue, Y.D., and Loke, W.H. (1997). Deficits in water escape performance and alterations in hippocampal cholinergic mechanisms associated with neonatal monosodium glutamate treatment in mice. *Pharmacol Biochem Behav*, 57(1-2): 383-388.

[17] Johnston, M.V. (1995). Neurotransmitters and vulnerability of the developing brain. *Brain and Development*, 17(5): 301-306.

[18] P. Offit. (2011) *Deadly Choices: How the Anti-Vaccine Movement Threatens Us All* (p. 178). New York: Basic Books.

[19] Kazmi, Z., Fatima, I., Perveen, S., and Malik, S.S. (2017). Monosodium glutamate: Review on clinical reports. *International Journal of Food Properties*, 20(5): 1807-1815,

[20] Ibid.

[21] Ibid.

Glyphosate—It's everywhere

"Vaccines, I would argue, are the best, safest things we put into our body. Obviously nothing is absolutely safe."

~Dr. Paul Offit, MD. *(Chief of the Division of Infectious Diseases).*

It's a fact that vaccines include contaminants. One of these contaminants (in the vaccine) can affect the glutamate functions in our brain. This would be glyphosate, the controversial active agent in *RoundUp*. Its use in weed-killing is how it made its way into vaccines. Animals eat food contaminated or altered by *RoundUp*. Parts of these animals are then used directly or indirectly in the manufacturing of vaccines.

In order to understand why glyphosate is dangerous to our body, we need to understand how it works. Glyphosate is detrimental to the Shikimate pathway. This pathway is found in plants and microorganisms such as bacteria. It's not found in human cells. One of this pathway's important functions is to combine aromatic compounds, such as aromatic acids and certain vitamins.[1]

As just mentioned, human cells don't contain the Shikimate pathway. So even though the aromatic acids are extremely important to us, our cells are not able to produce these acids. This is why the importance of getting them in our food is often stressed.[2]

Although human cells don't have the Shikimate pathway, our vast number of gut bacteria do. We are therefore reliant on our gut bacteria to produce these aromatic amino acids for us.

There hasn't been a lot of research on glyphosate in direct relation to vaccines, but there have been numerous studies on its effect on the

Shikimate Pathway. Several studies have found that glyphosate can cause oxidative stress.[34] Oxidative stress, which is also caused by glutamate, if you recall, is the product left over from free radical vs. antioxidant balance.

Ideally, this balance will even out and not result in oxidative stress. Oxidative stress is when we have an overabundance of free radicals damaging our cells. What makes a free radical dangerous is the fact that it's missing an electron, so it bounces around searching for one. In the meantime, it's causing damage and creating even more free radicals. This type of damage disrupts the mitochondria in our cells and has been linked to cancers[5] and many diseases.[67]

Everybody has it

Studies show that "glyphosate is detectable in around 90% of the US population."[8] So why do we care that we are injected with trace amounts of it in our vaccines? It's not like the vaccines are being digested in our gut where they can harm our bacterial environment. But keep in mind some of the chemicals in the vaccines enable them to travel freely through the gut-brain barrier and the blood-brain barrier.

Since glyphosate isn't really a vaccine ingredient, but rather a contaminant, how does it enter vaccines in the first place? Think about what vaccine viruses are grown in. The medium often consists of some type of animal source:

> "Contamination may come through bovine protein, bovine calf serum, bovine casein, egg protein and/or gelatin."[9]

Some vaccines contain gelatin, which is made from the bones and ligaments from farm animals such cows and pigs. And what have these animals likely been fed? Food like corn that has been treated with *RoundUp*. What is the active ingredient in *RoundUp*? Glyphosate.

When gelatin is used in vaccines, it very likely comes from animals which have been fed glyphosate-treated food. When gelatin is used in live viral vaccines, the virus can take the genetic coding from the glyphosate and incorporate it into its own genetic material. This can lead to autoimmune disease.[10]

Another way for glyphosate to cause autoimmune disease is once it has been injected into your body, it will contaminate your proteins and make them difficult to break down. This causes your immune system to create antibodies against the proteins the glyphosate has attached itself to. Now you have created antibodies against your own proteins and you start attacking your own cells. You now have the perfect potential for autoimmune diseases.

A test was performed on "nineteen different vaccines, from five manufacturers" for the presence of glyphosate. It's difficult to comprehend how glyphosate can even be detectable in vaccines considering the small role it plays in vaccine manufacturing. But in the Hepatitis B vaccine production process, for instance, genetically engineered yeast cells:

> *"[...] carry the surface antigen of the hepatitis B virus. The procedures result in a product that [...] could be a source of glyphosate if the yeast is grown on broths or media that utilize glyphosate-contaminated nutrient sources such as animal or plant proteins."*[11]

Of the 19 vaccines they tested, the vaccine that had the most glyphosate was the MMR II vaccine by Merck.

Both sugar beets and cow's milk are contaminated with glyphosate. Keep this in mind when reading the ingredients of the medium (where the germ is grown). Think of yeast, for instance. The yeast needs to be living and therefore the medium is given nutrients[12] to keep it alive. These include nutrients such as galactose and glucose, or in simple terms, milk and sugar. The glucose being the sugar source and galactose is from the lactose in the milk.

The above paper says the MMR vaccine contained the most glyphosate, why is that?

> *"This vaccine uses up to 12% hydrolysed gelatin as an excipient–stabilizer; as well as foetal bovine serum albumin, human serum albumin and residual chick embryo; all of which are contaminated by glyphosate during animal production."*[13]

Monsanto realized that glyphosate kills bacteria, so, in 2010, they patented glyphosate as an antimicrobial.[14] The list of pathogens affected by glyphosate is very long. What needs to be considered also is the fact that bacterium that's a pathogen in one part of the body is not necessarily a pathogen in another part of the body. Glyphosate doesn't discriminate between the two.

The most common hospital-acquired bacteria, *Pseudomonas aeruginosa*, can break down glyphosate. When it breaks it down, formaldehyde is produced.

Working together

Glyphosate actually blocks your cells from absorbing glutamate, so now you'll have a bunch of glutamate floating around in the space outside the cells. As you now know from the previous chapter, this causes excitotoxicity and oxidative stress.[15]

As a matter of fact, it has been shown that glyphosate "damages DNA and is a driver of mutations that lead to cancer."[16] This statement is based on using the US government GE crop data to find connections between glyphosate and 22 diseases, including stroke, diabetes, obesity, Alzheimer's disease (AD), autism and multiple sclerosis (MS). This study also answers the question of how on earth crops can survive glyphosate while it's killing everything else around it.

The researchers explain how they found genes in a bacterium that tolerates glyphosate. This gene was extracted and inserted into crop genes. Then the crops and their surroundings were covered in glyphosate. The crops, weeds and whatever else may be in the targeted area absorbed the glyphosate. Everything died except the crops because they had been injected with glyphosate-tolerant gene. [17]

Researchers from universities in Germany and Egypt collected blood and urine samples from dairy cows in Denmark. The purpose was to observe the presence of glyphosate and how it affects other markers such as those for the liver and its effect on important minerals such as manganese and zinc.[18] The researchers visited eight separate farms in Denmark and retrieved samples from 30 cows on each farm. All the cows tested positive for glyphosate.

In their discussion, the authors comment:

"It is amazing that more papers are not published about glyphosate excretion by farm animals since there are many papers reporting the detection of glyphosate in urine of humans, mostly of farmers using this herbicide."[19]

Regarding the blood samples taken from the cows, the results, say the authors "point to livers, kidneys and muscles damage." The authors continue explaining the behavior of glyphosate on nutrients:

"The glyphosate molecule grabs on to vital nutrients so they are not physiologically available. This process is called chelation and was actually the original property for which glyphosate was patented in 1964."[20]

The authors continue explaining that it wasn't until a decade later, in 1974, that it was used as an herbicide on crops. The authors' concerns regarding chelation is noticed towards the end of their paper where they explain:

"When applied to crops, glyphosate deprives them of vital minerals necessary for healthy plant function[...]. This also happens after ingestion of glyphosate in the body of animals and humans. Deficiency in trace elements like Mn, Cu, Zn, Se, Co, B, and Fe as well as macro elements like Mg, Ca, and others occur. Deficiencies of these elements in diets, alone or in combination, are known to interfere with vital enzyme systems and cause disorders and diseases."[21]

One year later, the authors of the above papers, together with other researchers, performed another study. This time they set out to test not just dairy cows, but also "hares, rabbits and humans." German researchers show when glyphosate containing crops is digested, the urine will test positive for glyphosate.[22]

Something we found interesting and even surprising, was that the "[f]armers who did not use rubber gloves had five times more glyphosate in their urine." Sounds like what they are saying is that you don't necessarily have to ingest (or be injected with) glyphosate to be contaminated, that it's enough to be in contact with it and it'll be absorbed through the skin.

In addition to testing humans for the presence of glyphosate, the authors also compared the results between those who are *chronically ill* with those who are *healthy*. The first mentioned had far more glyphosate in their urine than the latter.[23]

This wasn't just a concern of German scientists. In 2014, there was an analysis performed by scientists in America on the correlation between glyphosate and 22 diseases that seem to be continuously on the rise.

Although all 22 diseases were highly correlated, the diseases with the highest correlation with glyphosate were senile dementia (R=0.994), autism (R=0.989), thyroid cancers (R=0.988) and bladder cancer (R=0.981).[24] The "R" stands for *correlation coefficient* and has a value of -1.0 to + 1.0. The way this works is a negative value shows a negative relationship between the factors being compared. The factors in this case are glyphosate and various diseases. If the value is 0, it means there is no relationship at all between the factors, and a positive value shows a positive relationship between the factors being compared.

So, when you look at the correlation the authors found between glyphosate and dementia (R=0.994), you can see it is very close to 1.0, which is a near perfect relationship between the two.

The authors explain that glyphosate is toxic to our liver at as low as five parts per million (ppm). Even worse is it started messing with the glands that secrete hormones into our blood at 0.5 ppm. According to EPA in 2013 the maximum residual allowed in cattle was 5 ppm, and grain and cereal had a maximum residual allowance of 30 ppm.[25]

Another paper showed additional strong links between glyphosate and such diseases as "head and face anomalies [...], newborn eye disorders, newborn blood disorders, [...] new born skin disorders" and many more[26].

Stranger danger

A 'hazard assessment' by the World Health Organization's (WHO) International Agency for Research on Cancer (IARC) was released in March 2015 stating that glyphosate is "probably carcinogenic to humans."[27]

Hugh Grant, the Chairman of the Board of Directors and Chief Executive Officer at Monsanto, a Fortune 500 company, assures us in their sustainability report that:

> "At Monsanto, we're committed to [...] helping to take care of our planet, our people and the communities where we live and work."[28]

According to the Monsanto's webpage, an article written April, 2017, states that:

> "[...] regulatory agencies have reviewed all the key studies examined by IARC – and many more – and arrived at the overwhelming consensus that glyphosate poses no unreasonable risks to humans or the environment when used according to label instructions."[29]

Monsanto also state that: "no regulatory agency in the world considers glyphosate a carcinogen."[30] They also quote and link to agencies all over the world, stating that glyphosate does not pose a great risk to humans.

What if glutamate comes in contact with other chemicals, like aluminum? A study on exactly that was done in 2015. The paper explains how "Glyphosate disrupts gut bacteria." One example being *Clostridium difficile,* a bacterium that causes diarrhea, is given the opportunity to grow in abundance. This bacterium releases a toxin which boosts the aluminum to actions leading to anemia. Anemia is when red blood cells are either unable to carry normal amounts of oxygen, or there aren't enough red blood cells to carry the necessary amount of oxygen. As a result, we will suffer from hypoxia (lack of oxygen). This forces the pineal gland to make transferrin, which is an oxygen transporter on the red blood cell.

Aluminum, like so many other toxins involved in the vaccine manufacturing process, causes aluminum excitotoxicity.[31] This can be problematic for some individuals when glyphosate attaches itself to aluminum and helps it cross over both the gut-brain barrier and the blood-brain barrier (BBB).[32] The aluminum is no longer just causing problems in our blood stream, but also in the brain and gut.

Glyphosate also cloaks aluminum so it looks like calcium (Ca). This confuses the body in thinking glyphosate-aluminum compound is calcium. So, instead of absorbing calcium, the bones are absorbing glyphosate-aluminum compound. This can lead to the calcification of the pineal gland.

Besides making transferrin for oxygen transport, the pineal gland also produces melatonin. If we don't receive enough melatonin during the first few weeks after birth, there's a likelihood we'll have delayed mental process in performing motor movements.[33]

Chapter 20: Glyphosate – It's everywhere

[1] Dewick, P.M. (2001). *Medicinal Natural Products: A Biosynthetic Approach* (p. 121-166). England: John Wiley & Sons, ltd.

[2] Mir, R., Jallu, S., and Singh, T.P. (2015). The shikimate pathway: Review of amino acid sequence, function and three-dimensional structures of the enzymes. *Crit Rev Microbio*, 41(2): 172-189.

[3] Ahsan, N., Lee, D.G., Lee, K.W., Alam, I., Lee, S.H., Bahk, J.D., and Lee, B.H. (2008). Glyphosate-induced oxidative stress in rice leaves revealed by proteomic approach. *Plant Physiology and Biochemistry*, 46(12), 1062-1070.

[4] Chaufan, G., Coalova, I., and Rios de Molina Mdel, C. (2014). Glyphosate Commercial Formulation Causes Cytotoxicity, Oxidative Effects, and Apoptosis on Human Cells: Differences With its Active Ingredient. *Int J Toxicol*, 33(1): 29-38.

[5] Dreher, D. and Junod, A.F. (1996). Role of oxygen free radicals in cancer development. *Eur J Cancer*, 32A(1): 30-38.

[6] Bankson, D.D., Kestin, M., and Rifai, N. (1993). Role of free radicals in cancer and atherosclerosis. *Clin Lab Med*, 13(2): 463-480.

[7] Pham-Huy, L.A., He H., and Pham-Huy. C. (2008). Free Radicals, Antioxidants in Disease and Health. *International Journal of Biomedical Science*, 4(2): 89–96.

[8] *In Defence of Scientific Integrity: Examining the IARC Monograph Programme and Glyphosate Review,* Committee on Science, Space, and Technology House of Representatives, 115th Cong. 15 (2018). Retrieved from www.docs.house.gov/meetings/SY/SY00/20180206/106828/HHRG-115-SY00-20180206-SD004.pdf

[9] Samsel, A. and Seneff. S. (2017). Glyphosate pathways to modern diseases VI: Prions, amyloidoses and autoimmune neurological diseases. *Journal of Biological Physics and Chemistry*, 8-32.

[10] Ibid.

[11] Ibid.

[12] Broach, J.R. (2012). Nutritional Control of Growth and Development in Yeast. *Genetics*, 192(1), 73–105.

[13] Samsel, A. and Seneff. S. (2017). Glyphosate pathways to modern diseases VI: Prions, amyloidoses and autoimmune neurological diseases. *Journal of Biological Physics and Chemistry*, 8-32.

[14] Abraham, W. (n.d.). *Glyphosate formulations and their use for the inhibition of 5-enolpyruvylshikimate-3-phosphate synthase.* Retrieved from www.patents.google.com/patent/US7771736

[15] Cattani, D., de Liz Oliveira Cavalli, V.L., Heinz Rieg, C.E., Domingues, J.T., Dal-Cim, T., Tasca, C.I., and Zamoner, A. (2014). Mechanisms underlying the neurotoxicity induced by glyphosate-based herbicide in immature rat hippocampus: Involvement of glutamate excitotoxicity. *Toxicology*, 320: 34-45.

[16] Swanson, N.L., Leu, A., Abrahamson, J., and Wallet, B. (2014). Genetically engineered crops, glyphosate and the deterioration of health in the United States of America. *Journal of Organic Systems*, 9(2).

[17] Samsel, A. and Seneff. S. (2017). Glyphosate pathways to modern diseases VI: Prions, amyloidoses and autoimmune neurological diseases. *Journal of Biological Physics and Chemistry*, 8-32.

[18] Kruger, M., Schrödl, W., Neuhaus, J. and Shehata, A.A. (2013). Field Investigations of glyphosate in urine of danish dairy cows. *Journal of Environmental and Analytical Toxicology*, 3(5), 186-192.

[19] Ibid.

[20] Ibid.

[21] Ibid.

[22] Kruger, M., Schledorn, P., Schrödl, W., Hoppe, H-W., Lutz, W., and Shehata, A.A. (2014). Detection of glyphosate residues in animals and humans. *Journal of Environmental and Analytical Toxicology*, 4(2), 210-215.

[23] Ibid.

[24] N. Swanson, N.L., Leu, A.F., Abrahamson, J., and Wallet, B.C. (2014). Genetically engineered crops, glyphosate and the deterioration of health in the United States of America. *Journal of Organic Systems*, 9(2).

[25] Ibid. (Table 1).

[26] Hoy, J., Swanson, N., and Seneff, S. (2015). The High Cost of Pesticides: Human and Animal Diseases. *Poult Fish Wildl Sci*, 3:132.

[27] International Agency for Research on Cancer (IARC). (2018, January 03). *IARC Monograph on Glyphosate*. Retrieved from www.iarc.fr/featured-news/media-centre-iarc-news-glyphosate/

[28] Monsanto (2017). *Growing Better Together*. [Sustainability report]. Retrieved from www.monsanto.com/app/uploads/2017/12/Sustainability_2017.pdf

[29] Monsanto (February 12). *Response to Benbrook's Paper "Trends in Glyphosate Herbicide Use in the United States and Globally"*. Retrieved from www.monsanto.pr/response-to-benbrooks-paper-trends-in-glyphosate-herbicide-use-in-the-united-states-and-globally/

[30] www.monsanto.com/app/uploads/2017/12/Sustainability_2017.pdf

[31] Mundy, W.R.., Freudenrich, T.M., and Kodavanti, P.R. (1997). Aluminum potentiates glutamate-induced calcium accumulation and ironinduced oxygen free radical formation in primary neuronal cultures. *Mol. Chem. Neuropathol*, 32(1-3): 41-57.

[32] Seneff, S., Swanson, N. and Li, C. (2015). Aluminum and Glyphosate Can Synergistically Induce Pineal Gland Pathology: Connection to Gut Dysbiosis and Neurological Disease. *Agricultural Sciences*, 6(1): 42-70.

[33] Tauman, R., Zisapel, N., Laudon, M., Nehama, H., and Sivan, Y. (2002). Melatonin production in infants. *Pediatr Neurol*, 26(5):379-382.

CHAPTER 21

Glyphosate—Golden slumber

"Sleep is the best meditation."

~Dalai Lama.

Sleep is very important to human health. Stephanie Seneff, a senior research scientist at the Massachusetts Institute of Technology (MIT)[1], explains that in order for us to get good sleep, we need "to clear cellular debris."[2]

In her presentation, Dr. Seneff explains how the pineal gland releases melatonin. The melatonin then enters the fluid in our brain and spinal cord. Melatonin puts us in REM sleep. Without the shikimate pathway, there is no melatonin because the shikimate pathway produces the precursor for melatonin.[3]

Dr. Seneff continues to explain how lack of REM sleep, together with a calcified pineal gland, has been linked to Alzheimer's disease (AD). The pineal gland makes it possible for us to clean up our cellular debris, but when it's calcified it doesn't function properly.[4]

Because the pineal gland is not protected by the blood-brain barrier (BBB), it's more vulnerable to aluminum and mercury toxicity. When aluminum accumulates inside the pineal gland, it hinders its ability to clean cellular debris.

Another example of glyphosate's ability to block the shikimate pathway's functions is its relationship with sulfate. Sulfate is metabolized by the shikimate pathway. When sulfate is being stored, it's called Taurine. When women are pregnant, they release Taurine to the fetus. Taurine is also found in breast milk "and it accumulates in the neonatal brain."[5] If the mother doesn't have enough Taurine to pass on to the child, it can lead to stunted growth in the child, the CNS doesn't develop properly and the child will have low tolerance for glucose as well.[6]

Sulfate helps take care of acetaminophen, aluminum and mercury in the body. Children with autism only have about "1/3 the normal level of free sulfate in blood stream."[7]

When a chemical that's not supposed to be there enters our body, the consequences can range from not being a big deal at all to being life threatening. Most healthy individuals are able to take care of incoming toxicity and everything works out fine or at least seems to work out fine. We don't always connect the dots to future illnesses. Then there are individuals who have some dysfunction in their biological makeup they may not even know about. These dysfunctions may not cause any harm until they're exposed to certain elements or toxins.

Two-faced

If glyphosate is so bad for us, why do we have so many research papers saying how great it is? A paper published in 2010, states that:

> "[...] glyphosate is a one in a 100-year discovery that is important for reliable global food production as penicillin is for battling disease."[8]

A study involving injecting rats with MSG was conducted to find out whether male and female rats reacted differently. The results indicated they did. Glutamate caused a "dysfunction" in the male rats' "sexual behavior" more so than in the female rats. This was "mainly due to CNS damage"[9].

This was also observed in another study that looked into "the effects of testosterone on neuronal injury."[10]

The conclusion was that the difference between male and female was:

> "sex differences in response to brain injury are partly due to the consequence of damaging effects of testosterone."[11]

Another paper argues that:

> "We must be careful not to rush to label glyphosate as excessively toxic to humans because when used properly

*and in proper quantities it is probably no more dangerous
and toxic than other effective herbicides on the market."*[12]

The same paper points out that Samsel and Seneff's paper on glyphosate[13] is not a reliable study and argues it contains among other things:

*"[...], disconnected correlations, and manipulation of
number and conditions that create an epidemiological
recipe for errors and nonvalid associations."*[14]

The paper concludes by saying that "we must establish factual cause and effect relationships, rather than promote fear mongering, food scares, and lawsuits."[15] And under *disclosures,* the author states he has:

*"[...] no conflict of interest, except as a consumer who has
used this product for many years in my yard and would
not like to see it banned unless glyphosate is found guilty
as charged, [...]."*[16]

This article is full of accusatory statements and written throughout in that tone. Without dismissing the content, it's difficult to respect the statements in such an article or even take it (the article) seriously. There's a way to disagree with other scientists without dragging their work through the mud. At the end of the article, a sub-article is attached which has statements from both Seneff and Samsel commenting on this attack.

There seems to be much controversy regarding the safety of glyphosate, not only amongst scientists, but also higher up the ladder. The disagreements continue with IARC's contradicting statement that glyphosate is "probably carcinogenic to humans."[17], and the *health risk assessment* by the EPA, which was released in December 2017 stating that "glyphosate is not likely to be carcinogenic to humans."[18] (IARC is WHO's International Agency for Research on Cancer).

Did the biological agent change? Did science change? How can they both be examining the same agent and reach opposite conclusions?

This is where science gets tricky and it's easy to manipulate theories to mold a pleasing conclusion. Wordplay can be very confusing and misleading. The *minority report* from the Congressional hearing in February 2018, which can be watched online,[19] explains it this way:

> *"According to IARC, a cancer 'hazard' is an agent that is capable of causing cancer under some circumstances, while a cancer 'risk' is an estimate of the carcinogenic effects expected from exposure to a cancer hazard."*[20]

We have read this statement a hundred times and it's still unclear, vague and misleading. Monsanto is not pleased with IARC's assessment. In the Congressional hearing, Monsanto was presented with:

> *"hundreds of pages of internal Monsanto e-mails, memorandums, and other records that clearly show Monsanto engaged in a decades-long concerted effort to fend off any evidence suggesting potential adverse human health effects from glyphosate and more recently to undermine IARC's findings. They ghost wrote scientific articles on glyphosate, established front groups to help amplify their anti-IARC message and scientific evidence they did not like, and they attempted to silence scientists who reached their conclusions questioning glyphosate's safety."*[21]

If you're interested in Monsanto, we highly recommend listening to the entire hearing, where the Committee on Science, Space & Technology:

> *"[...] describes some of the tactics Monsanto has used to control the public debate about glyphosate as well as the scientific studies that have been conducted to assess its potential harm. These efforts appear aimed at corrupting and disrupting any honest, thorough and complete scientific evaluation of glyphosate and its potential adverse impact on the public's health."*[22]

Understanding how all these additional ingredients in the vaccine play on each other in some way, makes it easy to see how they can become magnified when combined. So, if, for instance, you're measuring the amount of formaldehyde in the vaccine, you're not taking into account whether the body is producing or being introduced to formaldehyde in any other way.

We also find it difficult to know which papers are legit, but we feel the research showing how glyphosate affects our cells on so many levels is worthy of notice. Although the argument is that glyphosate doesn't affect human cells, through the research we did for this chapter it's evident to us that our gut bacteria, which contains the shikimate pathway, is vital to many of our functions, especially its co-operation with our pineal gland.

Chapter 21: Glyphosate – Golden slumber

[1] CSAIL. (2018, January 18). Stephanie Seneff. Retrieved from www.csail.mit.edu/person/stephanie-seneff

[2] Seneff, S. (2014, March). *A Role for the Pineal Gland in Neurological Damage Following Aluminum-adjuvanted Vaccination.* [Power Point presented at the International Symposium on Vaccines, Nice, France]. Retrieved from www.people.csail.mit.edu/seneff/SeneffNice2014.pdf

[3] Ibid.

[4] Ibid.

[5] Seneff, S. (2018, March) *Sulfate is the most common nutritional deficiency that you never heard of.* [Power Point presentation in Toronto, Ontario Canada]. Retrieved from www.people.csail.mit.edu/seneff/2018/Toronto.pdf

[6] Ibid.

[7] Ibid.

[8] Powles, S.B. (2010). Gene Amplification Delivers Glyphosate-Resistant Weed Evolution. *Proc Natl Acad Sci U.S.A*, 107, 955–956.

[9] Sun, Y.M., Hsu, H.K., Lue, S.I., and Peng, M.T. (1991). Sex-specific impairment in sexual and ingestive behaviors of monosodium glutamate-treated rats. *Physiol Behav*, 50(5), 873-880.

[10] Yang, S.H., et al. (2002). Testosterone increases neurotoxicity of glutamate in vitro and ischemia-reperfusion injury in an animal model. *J Appl Physiol*, 92(1), 195-201.

[11] Ibid.

[12] Faria, M.A. (2015). Glyphosate, Neurological Diseases – and the Scientific Method. *Surg Neurol Int*, 6, 132.

[13] Samsel, A. and Seneff, S. (2015). Glyphosate, Pathways to Modern Diseases III: Manganese, Neurological Diseases, and Associated Pathologies. *Surg Neurol Int*, 6, 45.

[14] Faria, M.A. (2015). Glyphosate, Neurological Diseases – and the Scientific Method. *Surg Neurol Int*, 6, 132.

[15] Ibid.

[16] Ibid.

[17] *In Defence of Scientific Integrity: Examining the IARC Monograph Programme and Glyphosate Review,* Committee on Science, Space, and Technology House of Representatives, 115th Cong. 15 (2018). www.docs.house.gov/meetings/SY/SY00/20180206/106828/HHRG-115-SY00-20180206-SD004.pdf

[18] Ibid.

[19] Committee on Science, Space, & Technology. (2018, February 6). *Full Committee Hearing - In Defense of Scientific Integrity: Examining the IARC Monograph Programme and Glyphosate Review.* Retrieved from www.science.house.gov/legislation/hearings/full-committee-hearing-defense-scientific-integrity-examining-iarc-monograph

---

[20] *In Defence of Scientific Integrity: Examining the IARC Monograph Programme and Glyphosate Review,* Committee on Science, Space, and Technology House of Representatives, 115th Cong. 15 (2018).
www.docs.house.gov/meetings/SY/SY00/20180206/106828/HHRG-115-SY00-20180206-SD004.pdf
[21] Ibid.
[22] Ibid.

Prions & nanobacterium—Do you see me now?

*"Think of the earth as a living organism that
is being attacked by billions of bacteria whose
numbers double every forty years. Either the host
dies, or the virus dies, or both die."*

~**Gore Vidal** *(American writer)*

Among the contaminants that perhaps appear to be more concerning than any others are the tiny particles we don't know to test for. These particles sneak through the filtering process because they are so small, and they go undetected into the vaccines. Because we don't always know how to test for them, we don't even know they're there or whether or not they cause harm. And if they do, evidently, we don't know the severity of the harm.

Yet knowing this, the vaccines are still considered by some to be safe.

Prions

Prions are non-living proteins that cause the brain to die. They are known to be transmitted by eating the brain or nerve tissue from animals or humans infected by prions. This is normally called bovine spongiform encephalopathy (BSE), or mad cow disease in animals and transmissible spongiform encephalopathy (TSE) in humans.

The body is unable to defend itself against prions. This is because the prions are so small the body doesn't realize they're present and therefore fails to alert the immune system.

Since prions are not living organisms, but rather tiny pieces of proteins, it's impossible to kill them, regardless of temperature, toxins or other factors we use to make the attempt.

Because prions are not living, they don't have the ability to reproduce. Rather, they find a living cell and make copies of themselves. They don't go hunting for hosts because there's nothing driving them to do so. They are just protein fragments.

Interestingly, when these protein particles enter our body, the body reacts to them and starts making antibodies. But when we make vaccines out of chopped up proteins, we add adjuvants to aggravate the immune system because it doesn't recognize protein units on its own.

A paper written by the Department of Basic Pharmaceutical Sciences at University of South Carolina, US, states:

> "[...] hypothesized that various forms of prion diseases are essentially autoimmune diseases, resulting from chronic autoimmune attack of the central nervous system."[1]

Their hypothesis was strongly "supported by an overwhelming body of experimental observations that are scattered in the biomedical literature."[2]

Nano dose

The smallest bacteria we know of today are nanobacteria. These bacteria are so small they are able to pass through filters used in vaccine manufacturing. Not only that, they can also change their shape. When three lots of an inactivated polio vaccine were tested, two of them were positive for the presence of nanobacteria.

The Author of a paper from 1998 about contamination in cell cultures states that:

> "Large-scale cell culture operations for biotechnology products use millions of litres of complex media and gases as well as huge quantities of organic and inorganic raw materials. These raw materials must always be assumed to contain contamination by adventitious agents [...]."[3]

In 1985, an upper limit was determined on how much residual DNA could be in each vaccine dose. This limit was set by the FDA, the WHO and the European Medicines Agency (EMEA). The limit was 10 pg/dose. Later, in 1996, they determined they could have much more residual DNA without it causing any harm. They increased the limit to 10 ng/dose. This new limit did not include oral vaccines or vaccines from "microbial, diploid or primary cell cultures."[4]

After some further research, they decided that:

> *"[...] further data for DNA from continuous mammalian cell lines suggest it poses less risk than previously thought. For live viral vaccines or less purified products [...], it may not be possible to comply with the upper limit of the total DNA, i.e. 10 ng per dose."*[5]

The reason for being concerned enough about residual DNA to come up with an upper limit in the first place, is because there have been many studies on the safety of DNA fragments. The same paper states:

> *"[...] number of studies raised potential safety issues with regard to residual DNA. Residual DNA from continuous mammalian cell lines may transfer activated oncogenes and infectious provirus DNA."*[6]

There you have it. Residual DNA is known to be cancerous and includes infectious proviruses.

As with anything else that enters our body, be it vaccines or other substances, we don't understand how there can be such a thing as a safe amount. Two children of the same age can sit at the same table, one eating a sandwich and the other in danger of dying from ingesting as much as a bread crumb.

It is impossible to determine the maximum amount of a substance one child or infant can have based on the amount given to another child. We see evidence of this every day in our daily lives. Let's take 20 kindergartners for instance. It's the first day of school and they're all playing together in the same classroom. Some will come home sick while others won't. We're not saying this is the same thing, we are merely pointing out that humans can react very differently even when exposed to the exact same environment.

Pigs and yeast in vaccines

Other proteins of concern are from pigs and yeast. Besides allergic reactions, many people have shown religious concerns regarding vaccines and their ingredients. Muslims and the use of gelatin (pig) being a case in point. Because of this, representatives from various religions have been consulted.

In regards to Kashrut or Jewish kosher dietary laws:

> "according to Jewish laws, there is no problem with porcine or other animal derived ingredients in non-oral products. This includes vaccines, including those administered via the nose, injections, suppositories, creams and ointments."[7]

The article also mentions:

> "In 2001, the World Health Organization (WHO) consulted with over 100 Muslim scholars and confirmed that the gelatin used is considered halal and there is no religious reason not to receive vaccination."[8]

There are many shortcomings regarding ethical use of vaccine ingredients. These range from using aborted fetal cells to using porcine proteins. It's almost impossible to create a product that satisfies all belief systems so we cannot blame scientists for not being able to accommodate everyone.

A more important question would be whether there should be exemptions for people of different religious persuasions. We will not discuss the ethics of vaccine usage relating to different belief systems as we feel that would be a book on its own. Anyway, it's each to his or her own as far as we are concerned.

Chapter 22: Prions & nanobacterium – Do you see me now?

[1] Zhu, B.T. (2005). Human and animal spongiform encephalopathies are the result of chronic autoimmune attack in the CNS: a novel medical theory supported by overwhelming experimental evidence. *Histol Histopathol*, 20(2), 575-592.

[2] Ibid.

[3] Garnick, R.L. (1998). Raw materials as a source of contamination in large-scale cell culture. *Dev Biol Stand*, 93, 21-29.

[4] World Health Organization, Quality Assurance and Safety of Biologicals. (2005, April). *Report of the WHO Informal consultation on the application of molecular methods to assure the quality, safety and efficacy of vaccines*. Retrieved from: www.who.int/biologicals/Molecular%20Methods%20Final%20Mtg%20Report%20April2005.pdf?ua=1

[5] Ibid.

[6] Ibid.

[7] Public Health England. (2013). "Porcine content in vaccines: faith communities and people with dietary restrictions." *Vaccine update*. 206. Retrieved from: www.assets.publishing.service.gov.uk/government/uploads/system/uploads/attachment_data/file/244730/vaccine_update_206_19_9.pdf

[8] Ibid.

CHAPTER 23

Mycoplasma—It's a sticky situation

"The only safe vaccine is one that is never used."

~Dr. James A. Shannon, MD, *Former Director, National Institutes of Health (1955–1968)*

One of the most common and notorious contaminants plaguing vaccine manufacturers is other bacteria. Laboratories do test for some bacteria, but not all are detected, especially if they are fastidious or slow-growing and therefore not detectible until late in the process. In this chapter, we are only going to mention one of them: mycoplasma.

There are multiple ways mycoplasma ends up in vaccines during the manufacturing stage. This bacterium is everywhere and it requires a good imagination to think of all the ways mycoplasma infiltrates the vaccine-making process. The opportunities are not isolated to locations inside the lab as the bacterium can easily be brought in via vents, humans or whatever else enters the lab.

According to a paper published in *Vaccine*, one of the reasons is plain and simple, lab hygiene:

> *"Mycoplasma contaminants can be considered important not only because of their role as pathogens but also because they may indicate that insufficient care has been taken during vaccine manufacture or quality control."*[1]

Mycoplasma can multiply undetected in the cell cultures and can grow even in presence of antibiotics.

Lab hopping

According to *Corning Incorporated* bulletin on 'Understanding and Managing Cell Culture Contamination,' there have been various studies on mycoplasma contamination in vaccine manufacturing across the world. For instance, in the Netherlands, "1949 cell cultures" were tested and 25% of them were positive for mycoplasma; in Czechoslovakia, 327 cell cultures were tested and 37% of them were positive for mycoplasma; in Argentina, 65% of the cell cultures tested positive; and in Japan, 80% of the cell cultures tested positive for mycoplasma.[2]

As the brochure explains, the problem often lies in the particles that are stirred into the air during laboratory work. These particles can be from the preparation of cell cultures, lab coats and other clothing, skin (especially from much handwashing), lab equipment (i.e. pipets), incubators, even the air flow hood. The sources are many. This can become even more complicated if animals are stored nearby.

Potentially, the bacteria can piggyback on lab technician errors as well. To show how simple mistakes can be made in the lab, resulting in serious consequences, the brochure gives these examples:

> "A technician retrieved a vial labeled WI-38 from a liquid nitrogen freezer thinking it contained the widely used diploid human cell line. once in culture, it was immediately discovered to be a plant cell line derived from a common strain of tobacco called Wisconsin 38, also designated WI-38.

> "Two separate research laboratories, both attempting to develop cell lines from primary cultures, shared a walk-in incubator. One lab used the acronyms HL-1, HL-2, etc. to identify the primary cultures they derived from human lung. The other lab worked with cultures derived from human liver, but they too (unknowingly) used the identical coding system. It wasn't long before a culture mix-up occurred between the two laboratories." [3]

It's one thing when mistakes are caught before the vaccines are distributed to the public.

But what about those times they are not recognized and no-one's aware that mistakes were made?

There appears to be enough toxic ingredients and unknown dangers packed into the solution we're injected with. It should be mandatory to fully inform us *before* we consent to be vaccinated or have our children vaccinated. Such knowledge would empower us to make more informed decisions affecting our health and our children's health.

To keep us in the dark on these dangers and force vaccination upon everyone feels highly unethical and undemocratic. To get a closer look at *forced* vaccinations, we visited a website for the vaccine schedules in EU countries[4]. It appears not all the countries in the European Union feel it's necessary to force vaccinations on their children 18 months or younger. We discovered that although all 31 countries recommend vaccinations, 20 don't mandate any of them. Surprisingly, some of the countries *don't* recommend the varicella vaccine. Only two (Italy and Latvia) mandate all the vaccines on the list (diphtheria, tetanus, pertussis, hepB, polio, hib, measles, mumps, rubella, varicella).

In order for children in all 50 states in the US to attend public schools, they are required to be vaccinated. That being said, some states have religious or philosophical exemptions.[5] Australia as well has mandated vaccines insomuch as they will not pay "Child Care Benefit (CCB) and Child Care Rebate (CCR) payments" because the Government is "extremely concerned at the risk non-vaccinated children pose to public health."[6]

For those who wish to hold off on certain vaccines, we recommend you look into the exemptions many countries offer, especially if you're concerned about the status of your child's immune system.

Chapter 23: Mycoplasma – It's a sticky situation

[1] Thornton, D.H. (1986). A survey of mycoplasma detection in veterinary vaccines. *Vaccine*. 4(4), 237-240.

[2] Ryan, J. (2012). *Understanding and Managing Cell Culture Contamination*. [Technical Bulletin]. N.Y. Corning Incorporated. Retrieved from:
www.safety.fsu.edu/safety_manual/supporting_docs/Understanding%20and%20Managing%20Cell%20Culture%20Contamination.pdf

[3] Ibid.

[4] European Centre for Disease Prevention and Control (ECDC). (n.d.). *Vaccine schedules in all countries of the European Union*. Retrieved from www.vaccine-schedule.ecdc.europa.eu/

[5] Skinner, E. (2017, Dec). A quick look into important issues of the day (Vol. 25, No 48). [LegisBrief]. Retrieved from
http://www.ncsl.org/documents/legisbriefs/2017/lb_2548.pdf

[6] Klapdor, M. and Grove, A. (n.d.). *'No Jab No Pay' and other immunisation measures*. [Budget Review 2015-26 Index]. Retrieved from
www.aph.gov.au/About_Parliament/Parliamentary_Departments/Parliamentary_Library/pubs/rp/BudgetReview201516/Vaccination

CHAPTER 24

Wrapping up Part One

"All things can be deadly to us, even the things made to serve us; as in nature walls can kill us, and stairs can kill us, if we do not walk circumspectly."

~Blaise Pascal, *Pensées*

Manufacturing vaccines can be a very complex procedure, requiring many different techniques, depending on the type of vaccine needed for certain diseases.

There is, for instance, as mentioned in an earlier chapter, a big difference depending on whether we are dealing with a bacterium or a virus. Bacteria can easily be grown in a nutritional growth media whereas viruses have to be grown in living cells. This is because bacteria are living organisms and viruses are not.

It's also important to remember that as with any other mass-produced substances (and objects), each batch may vary. Even though it's the same vaccine, some batches may be more contaminated than others. Examples of this will be mentioned in Part Two of this book. We will also highlight the fact that a disease can be caused by a germ that has multiple strains— another aspect of the production process.

It can be quite a challenge for scientists to know which strains to include in the vaccines.

Viruses are not considered living organisms and are unable to replicate without the help of a living host. It is therefore necessary to inject the vaccine virus into living cell cultures in order for it to make copies of itself. Therefore, many vaccines today are still being grown in live cell cultures. The cells contained in these cultures can contain thousands of different proteins and other substances that will cause our immune system to react.

So, when someone says the vaccine only contains one or two antigens, although maybe true in theory, it's *not* accurate when all the other components involved in the manufacturing process are taken into account.

We hope we have given you enough information to carry with you into Part Two of this book. In the coming chapters we will be highlighting some of the childhood vaccines and illnesses known to be associated with vaccines. Because there are so many variants of vaccines throughout the world, it would take a much bigger book to detail each and every one. We will therefore focus mostly on the ones which have the most accessible information, namely those vaccines on the CDC's childhood immunization schedule. We have, in addition, added a little table showing the various vaccines and their accompanying ingredients in appendix 1.

We urge you to connect the dots between *what you already knew* about vaccines and *what you now know* after reading Part One. And we hope you now understand how very, very difficult it is to link an illness or disorder to one specific vaccine or substance. In addition to vaccines, we are also simultaneously and constantly exposed to toxins via food, products or the very air we breathe.

PART TWO

Vaccines: the illnesses they are meant to protect and the illnesses they potentially create

CHAPTER 25

Diphtheria, tetanus & pertussis—Sudden death

*"Experiments to produce anaphylactic shock
are facilitated by addition of pertussis vaccine to
the solution: the mice (or rabbits, or hamsters, or
whatever) die more rapidly, and in larger
numbers. By the same token, addition of the
vaccine to the sterile brain and spinal cord
solution greatly enhances it's ability to generate
an allergic encephalitis."*

*~Harris Coulter, Vaccination, Social
Violence, and Criminality: The Medical Assault
on the American Brain*

Diphtheria, pertussis and tetanus (DTP) vaccine is a cocktail of toxoids in one single shot.

When the vaccine is being manufactured, it's actually manufactured as three separate vaccines: a diphtheria vaccine, a pertussis vaccine and a tetanus vaccine. After they have all been made, they are then combined into one single vial.

In the production process of the diphtheria vaccine, only the toxins are extracted from bacteria and used. The toxins inside *Corynebacterium diphtheriae* are proteins called exotoxins. These proteins help the bacterium grow. After the exotoxins finish their job they are released.

Unfortunately for we humans, when the exotoxins are released inside our body, they can be harmful. They destroy our cellular production of proteins and this eventually kills the cells.

When manufacturing the tetanus vaccine, the toxins from *Clostridium tetani, diphtheriae's* cousin, are extracted and used. These toxins enter our body when we puncture our skin, such as when we step on a rusty nail. Just like *diphtheriae*, *C. tetani* is harmless without its toxins. *C. tetani* produces two toxins, but we're only interested in the harmful one, tetanospasmin, which takes away our muscles' ability to relax by blocking nerve signals.

The third vaccine added to this triple combination vaccine is called *Bordetella pertussis*. This one behaves quite differently to the other two. Instead of utilizing exotoxins, it contains endotoxins. Endotoxins are an actual part of the cell wall. When the bacterium dies, the cell wall breaks and the toxins leak into the surrounding environment.

Pertussis has three components that can make us sick. One of them is the cyclase toxin (CyaA), which causes the infamous whopping cough. Another one is the pertussis toxin (PT toxin), which attacks the macrophages in our throat, and the last one is filamentous hemagglutinin (FHA). This one's a sticky son of a gun.

The sticky mucous substance, hemagglutinin, allows the bacteria stick to our mucosal lining. This makes it difficult to breathe, especially for a tiny baby with narrow airways.

Now let's think about this for a second and summarize what we know so far. When a natural infection occurs, the germ becomes trapped in our mucosal tissue where immunoglobulin A (IgA) antibodies attack and produce memory immunity. In a vaccine injection, these toxins are not entering the body via mucosal lining in its natural state within the bacteria. Rather, they are injected straight into the bloodstream as toxoids.

The death DTaP

We were surprised to see Sudden Infant Death Syndrome (SIDS) mentioned on a few of the package inserts. After some digging, we realized some argue SIDS is connected to the pertussis toxoids while others claim there are not enough cases to substantiate any such correlation.

One common adverse reaction, not only as a reaction to the DTaP vaccine, but many others as well, is apnea. Another one is cyanosis. So, we wondered whether this could be one of the many times where the wording confuses the consistency of diagnosis.

How would apnea and cyanosis be confused with SIDS? Apnea is the absence of breathing. Cyanosis occurs when the skin or tissues don't receive enough oxygen and turn blue. When a baby dies with its skin turning blue and/or not breathing could it be diagnosed with SIDS?

There are cases where apnea or cyanosis occur and is caught in time to resuscitate the baby (and baby survives). These cases will then, of course, not be counted as SIDS. Does that mean they shouldn't be a part of the statistics in the warning section of SIDS in adverse events? Aren't the symptoms of SIDS the same as a child with apnea or cyanosis up to the point of resuscitation?

The only reason someone needs to be resuscitated is because he or she ceased to breathe. Are we missing something? Is it safe to say that if a baby's death is attributed to apnea, it died from SIDS? If the baby's death is attributed to apnea and not SIDS, does that lower the SIDS deaths stats?

In the 1970s, Japan experienced multiple infant deaths claimed to be caused by the DPT vaccine. This was quite concerning for the Japanese Government. So, by making some adjustments to Eli Lily's own vaccine-recipe, they made a purer and safer acellular pertussis vaccine. Japan started using this new vaccine in 1981.

Although this incident was widely reported and well known, the US kept using the more reactive version of the vaccine. Not surprisingly, perhaps, by the mid-1980s in the US, the side-effects from the DTP vaccine had triggered about 300 lawsuits against the vaccine manufacturers.

Authors of another study, this one done in India, conclude that there is no association between SIDS and DTP vaccine. Something we found a little odd was that they exclude all the children who had "any history of risk of SIDS in family or to child"[1]. What makes us curious about this exclusion, is, would these children have been excluded from receiving vaccination if they were not a part of the study?

It seems to be a consistent flaw in study trial designs that they don't include those at higher risk in the test (vaccine) group. This, of course, makes sense, but it's also very misleading. It biases the study towards falsely high safety results.

A research paper on Infant Mortality Rates (IMR), states that 'Crib death,' which is another term for SIDS, used to be so unheard of. It wasn't even recorded in the 'infant mortality statistics'[2].

The authors continue:

> *"For the first time in history, most US infants were*
> *required to receive several doses of DPT, polio, measles,*
> *mumps, and rubella vaccines. Shortly thereafter, in 1969,*
> *medical certifiers presented a new medical term – sudden*
> *infant death syndrome. In 1973, the National Center for*
> *Health Statistics added a new cause-of-death category –*
> *for SIDS – to the ICD. [...] By 1980, SIDS had become the*
> *leading cause of postneonatal mortality (deaths of infants*
> *from 28 days to one year old) in the United States."*[3]

The authors also mention conclusions drawn in other research papers as well. For instance, they state that in Australia it was found "when the SIDS rate decreased, deaths attributed to asphyxia increased."[4]

Could this be another case of wide selection of diagnosis?

In the early 2000s, SIDS was replaced by diagnoses like 'suffocation in bed' and 'unknown causes.' Not surprisingly, less children suffered from SIDS after that.[5]

Although their study or conclusion isn't about whether the vaccines cause SIDS, they found that: "*nations that require more vaccine doses tend to have higher infant mortality rates.*"[6]

How safe do the FDA and the CDC feel this vaccine is? This question relates to a study that was funded by these two organizations. The conclusion of this study isn't necessarily their official standing on the matter. The authors used the Vaccine Adverse Event Reporting System (VAERS) to collect data on adverse events in relation to the DTaP vaccine from January 1, 1991 through December 31, 2016.[7]

The authors of the study were not surprised to find SIDS to be the most prevalent since SIDS is "the fourth leading cause of death in the United States among infants" and according to the Vaccine Safety Datalink (VSD), it's "the second leading cause of death among children aged 0 to 18 months."[8] They continue by explaining how the incidence of SIDS has actually gone down with time and don't believe the DTaP vaccine is the causal factor for SIDS.

Keep in mind that all cases of adverse events from vaccinations reported to the FDA are believed to be less than one percent of all actual cases.[9] Despite this, in a 15-year period, with less than one percent of adverse events reported, 844 deaths of children who received the DTaP vaccine were officially acknowledged. They also found official records for 725 of these deaths, which they categorized under *Cause of Death*. In their list of reasons, SIDS was highest with 350 deaths (48.3%). *Undetermined and Other* (causes) equaled 119 deaths (16.4%).

Their argument is that rather than it being the vaccine causing SIDS, it's merely a coincidental factor as it happens to be administered together with multiple other vaccines and at an age when children are most likely to die from SIDS.

Viral awakening

Apart from SIDS, there have been other incidences of death from this vaccine. As you may remember, formaldehyde (FA) is used to inactivate the toxins. It does this by randomly destroying some of the surface proteins. Unfortunately, because formaldehyde isn't coded for specific proteins, we have no idea which proteins it will break.

An incident involving the use of formaldehyde is the 1948 Kyoto Disaster in Japan. Some 606 children received a vaccine containing the diphtheria toxoid. Something happened during the manufacturing that caused the toxoid to 'wake up' and revert back to its original toxin. This caused 68 of the 606 children to die. That's more than 10%. Imagine if there had been hundreds of thousands of children vaccinated.

Authors of a paper that summarized a workshop on neurological effects of vaccines state:

> *"[...] there is sufficient experimental data to implicate both endotoxin and PT [pertussis toxin] in adverse neurologic reactions to pertussis vaccine."*[10]

In 2018, a paper on 'the Pertussis Enigma' the authors explain that:

> *"According to 2008 estimates, pertussis caused 16 million cases and 195 000 deaths in children younger than 5 years old worldwide, despite a global 82% vaccine coverage."*[11]

They continue:

> *"whole-cell and acellular pertussis (aP) vaccines do not protect against transmission and that waning of infection- or vaccine-derived immunity generates an endemic pool of adults, who act as a reservoir of transmission to young children."*[12]

The authors set out to look into the validity of these statements. They collected data from 32 countries, and only four (Australia, Israel, Netherlands, U.S.A) had increased incidences in pertussis from 1980 to 2012. The authors include graphs showing the 20 countries that switched from whole cell pertussis vaccine to the acellular pertussis vaccine, to see if there was a shift in incidence of disease. Interestingly, they were unable to find a solid answer.

The data is not consistent between all the countries. What seems to apply in one country doesn't necessarily apply in another.

Besides the four countries mentioned above (four countries which actually showed a steady incline in pertussis incidence), Italy had a drastic decrease in pertussis cases. South Korea continued to see a drop in cases after they switched over to acellular pertussis, but then suddenly, a decade later, the number of cases rose steadily.

The authors' overall conclusion, after reviewing all their data, is that there isn't enough consistency to draw even a hypothetical conclusion on the vaccine's behavior.[13]

We don't know if DTaP plays a role in SIDS, but we do find the circumstantial correlations undeniable. It would be interesting to pull the same data from other countries and compare their vaccine schedules with SIDS or similar infant deaths. Another aspect that would be interesting to look into is adding the vaccine brand used in each of these countries or cases.

Chapter 25: Diphtheria, tetanus & pertussis – Sudden death

[1] Srinivas, K., Preeti, G., and Pasula, S. (2015). DPT immunization and SIDS."*Int J Contemp Pediatr*, 2(3), 202-207.

[2] Miller, N.Z., and Goldman, G.S. (2011). Infant Mortality Rates Regressed against Number of Vaccine Doses Routinely given: Is There a Biochemical or Synergistic Toxicity? *Human & Experimental Toxicology*, 30(9), 1420–1428.

[3] Ibid.

[4] Ibid.

[5] Ibid.

[6] Ibid.

[7] Moro, P.L., Perez-Vilar, S., Lewis, P., Bryant-Genevier, M., Kamiya, H., and Cano, M. (2018). Safety Surveillance of Diphtheria and Tetanus Toxoids and Acellular Pertussis (DTaP) Vaccines. *Pediatrics*, 142(1).

[8] Ibid.

[9] Harvard Pilgrim Health Care, Inc. (n.d.). *Electronic Support for Public Health-Vaccine Adverse Event Reporting System (ESP:VAERS)*. [Grant final report]. Retrieved from: www.healthit.ahrq.gov/sites/default/files/docs/publication/r18hs017045-lazarus-final-report-2011.pdf

[10] Menkes, J.H. and Kinsbourne, M. (1990). Workshop on Neurologic Complications of Pertussis and Pertussis Vaccination. *Neuropediatrics*, 21(4), 171-176.

[11] Domenech de Cellès, M., Magpantay, F.M.G., King, A.A., and Rohani, P. (2016). The Pertussis Enigma: Reconciling Epidemiology, Immunology and Evolution. *Proc Biol Sci.* 283(1822), 20152309.

[12] Ibid.

[13] Ibid.

CHAPTER 26

Diphtheria, tetanus & pertussis—Controversy

*"Leave your drugs in the chemist's pot if you
can cure the patient with food."*

~Hippocrates (Greek physician 420 BC)

Another illness that has been associated with, among other vaccines, the DTaP vaccine, is Guillain-Barré Syndrome (GBS). It's said to be an autoimmune disorder caused by molecular mimicry.

Molecular mimicry is when invading antigens, like those in a vaccine, look a lot like our own proteins. This process starts when these invading particles activate our immune cells causing them to release cytokines to clean out invading germs or antigens. Cytokines are proteins that help cells communicate with each other by signaling certain commands and messages. So, in molecular mimicry, these cytokines, and other actions our body has initiated, start cleaning out their own antigens also, hence autoimmunity.

Another syndrome that has been associated with tetanus toxoid is antiphospholipid syndrome (APS). This happens when the body has too many antibodies (proteins) fighting the invading molecules.[1] It's an autoimmune disease where the body attacks our phospholipids. Phospholipids is fat inside our cells. Such an attack damages our cells and causes our blood to thicken and clot. This can have many complicated health problems, including heart attacks and kidney damage. Other factors that cause this syndrome are bacteria, viruses and yeast.[2] Needless to say, these are all vaccine ingredients as well. Sometimes this syndrome is called Hughes Syndrome.

What about the Shaken Baby Syndrome (SBS)? After a closer look this syndrome turned out to be more technical than expected. It's normally associated with its synonym pediatric abusive head trauma (AHT).

A chapter on this subject in *StatPearls,* defines SBS as:

> *"Abusive head trauma with a pattern of injuries that may include retinal hemorrhages and regular patterns of brain injury.*

> *"[...] used to describe brain injury symptoms consistent with vigorously shaking an infant or small child."*[3]

According to the National Institutes of Health (NIH), the Shaken Baby Syndrome (SBS) can be related to vaccines, including the DTaP vaccine. This has been linked with Barlow's disease, which is vitamin C deficiency in infants. Barlow's disease looks a lot like SBS and therefore has been mistaken for child abuse. [4]

This link between "Vaccine-induced vitamin C deficiency" and SBS was also acknowledge in Sweden in 2016.[5]

Shaken Baby Syndrome is often referred to in scientific literature as 'non-accidental injury.' Scientists have known for more than 80 years that the pertussis vaccine causes brain damage. The controversy isn't really over the fact that it happens, but how often it happens.

One thing, many names

Another adverse event DPT vaccine is said to trigger, are seizures. This is included in the package inserts. As with so many other disorders, seizures have gone through multiple labels. You will find some of them in the package inserts.

What if your child is diagnosed with infantile spasm? This disorder is not included in the package insert, yet it is a form of a seizure. We wondered whether these children were automatically included in the seizure category or if they were not counted at all.

Other labels include cerebral palsy, convulsions and epilepsy. We're aware these are all considered to be slightly different, but by dividing seizures into so many categories, does it make seizures as an adverse event look less frequent? Does it make a seizure appear to be a rare event when perhaps it isn't all that rare?

Sick with it

Another concern is the fact that the vaccine appears to have the ability to cause the diseases it's trying to protect us from. Whooping cough has re-emerged among those ailments vaccinated against all over the world.

A paper from 2016 states:

> *"[...] acellular vaccines, although protective against pertussis disease, do not protect against* B. pertussis *infection."*[6]

This means that you may not become sick, but you can still carry the bacteria in your body and infect others.

Another study suggests there are individuals who have been vaccinated and then catch the disease. They may not know they have it because the symptoms are not being expressed, but the bacteria are still present in their body. This way they become a walking reservoir for everyone around them.[7]

Chapter 26: Diphtheria, tetanus & pertussis -- Controversy

[1] National Human Genome Research Institute (NHGRI). (2010, Dec. 15th). Learning About Antiphospholipid Syndrome (APS). *National Human Genome Research Institute (NHGRI)*. Retrieved from: www.genome.gov/17516396/learning-about-antiphospholipid-syndrome/

[2] Cusick, M.F., Libbey, J.E., and Fujinami, R.S. (2012). Molecular Mimicry as a Mechanism of Autoimmune Disease. *Clin Rev Allergy Immunol*, 42(1), 102–111.

[3] Joyce, T., and Huecker, M.R. (2018). Pediatric Abusive Head Trauma (Shaken Baby Syndrome). In B. Abai, et al (Eds.). *StatPearls*. Retrieved from www.ncbi.nlm.nih.gov/books/NBK499836/#article-28960.s1

[4] Innis, M. (2006). Vaccines, Apparent Life-Threatening Events, Barlowís Disease, and Questions about 'Shaken Baby Syndrome'. *Journal of American Physicians and Surgeons*, 11(1), 17-19. Retrieved from: www.jpands.org/vol11no1/innis.pdf

[5] Swedish Agency for Health Technology Assessment and Assessment of Social Services (SBU). (2016). *Traumatic shaking – The role of the triad in medical investigations of suspected traumatic shaking*. [Systematic review]. Retrieved from www.sbu.se/contentassets/09cc34e7666340a59137ba55d6c55bc9/traumatic_shaking_2016.pdf

[6] Locht, C. (2016). Pertussis: Where did we go wrong and what can we do about it? *J Infect*, 72, S34-S40.

[7] Althouse, B.M. and Scarpino, S.V. (2015) Asymptomatic transmission and the resurgence of Bordetella pertussis. *BMC Med*, 13, 146.

CHAPTER 27

Bias

"Science is the search for truth, that is the effort to understand the world: it involves the rejection of bias, of dogma, of revelation, but not the rejection of morality."

~**Linus Pauling** *(American scientist).*

Dr. James D. Cherry[1] from New Jersey has a very impressive medical career, especially within the field of infectious diseases. He has performed studies funded by, among others, Sanofi Pasteur and GSK. In 2003 he received the Pediatric Infectious Disease Society Distinguished Physician Award.[2] Among Dr. Cherry's multiple studies on vaccine trials, he wrote one together with Stanley Plotkin[3] about the 'one-size-fits-all' bias used in data collection.[4]

In the paper the authors go on to explain how trials can be skewed by the fact that different countries have different case definitions for pertussis.

As an example, they state in the above paper that:

> *"France requires that cough be present for more than 7 days, whereas Australia accepts cough of any duration if it is accompanied by paroxysms, whooping, or vomiting. The EU also accepts any physician's diagnosis of pertussis and apnea as a clinically defining symptom in infants."*[5]

Their major concern is that pertussis is not being diagnosed often enough, which means the vaccine usage will not increase:

> *"Without knowing that the disease predominantly occurs in this population, attempts to increase vaccine use in adolescents and adults are unlikely to be made."*[6]

199

It's perhaps not a surprise this was funded by Sanofi Pasteur. Either way, it shows that misdiagnosing can be a concern for both vaccine manufacturers and those expressing concerns over vaccine safety.

In another paper written by J.D Cherry in 2011, he expresses concern about the 2010 pertussis epidemic in California. The media attributed the epidemic to vaccine failures. When Dr. Cherry took a closer look, he determined the vaccine did not live up to its expectations due to case definition. [7]

Eventually, the World Health Organization (WHO) came up with a standardized case definition. The author, J.D Cherry, in his above-mentioned paper, shares something that surprised us a little:

> *"I was a member of the WHO committee and disagreed with the primary case definition because it was clear at that time that this definition would eliminate a substantial number of cases and therefore inflate reported efficacy values."* [8]

Which must surely raise the question if you are a vaccine researcher receiving funding from vaccine manufacturers, should you be on the WHO committee that determines the case definition? Maybe this is normal, we haven't looked into it, but it just seems like conflict of interest.

There appear to be multiple biases in play when it comes to data collected for vaccine trials included in the package inserts. These include concerns such as when researchers interview parents or guardians to gather data and when researchers cherry-pick healthy individuals to participate in their vaccine trials. The latter is called Healthy User Bias (HUB). The end result being, of course, the vaccinated group will consist of stronger and healthier individuals.

A paper on HUB in a DPT vaccine study on SIDS reported in 1992 that, to reconfirm what we said above, those who have a predisposition for SIDS or encephalopathy would not be given the vaccine for the study. Therefore, it doesn't represent the actual risk of the vaccine. [9] Instead, these individuals are put in the unvaccinated group, which makes this group unfairly prone to illness or death.

In a nutshell, as we understand it, the authors of the study are expressing concerns that the study design is excluding the very people who are prone to adverse effects potentially triggered or caused by the vaccine.

In their concluding remarks, they state:

"The fact that such biases do exist makes it difficult to demonstrate convincingly that a vaccine is not responsible for rare, severe, adverse reactions."[10]

The WHO published a review on several DTP vaccine studies and infant deaths. They found the studies were designed or performed in a biased and inconsistent manner.[11]

Another concern to look out for is the fact that predisposed children may not be excluded from the study. Meaning, instead of being put in the vaccinated group, they are put in the group which does not receive the DTP vaccine. But since these children are already fragile, they are more prone to illnesses or even death. These two groups are then compared to each other.

Then authors of a paper published in 2017 discussed observations made in multiple studies on frailty and survival biases.[12] Another study by some of the same authors echoes the sentiment when they state that "[m]ost observations were repeated in several studies and generated new deductions"[13]. So, not only is the formerly biased data used to draw a conclusion, but it is then re-used for multiple studies. Studies which use the data for their own interpretations.

Perhaps the statement that stood out the most to us in the above-mentioned study was when the authors suggested that:

"All currently available evidence suggests that DTP vaccine may kill more children from other causes than it saves from diphtheria, tetanus or pertussis. Though a vaccine protects children against the target disease it may simultaneously increase susceptibility to unrelated infections."[14]

Gender discrimination

Another observation the authors made was that vaccinated girls had a considerably higher mortality rate than vaccinated boys. This ratio was highly dependent on whether or not the oral polio vaccine (OPV) was given simultaneously. For instance, girls receiving the DPT were 12 times more likely to die than unvaccinated girls. But if the OPV was given simultaneously, the vaccinated girls were 9.5 times more likely to die than the unvaccinated girls.

Compare this to the boys, and the difference is surprising. The boys receiving DPT vaccine by itself were 8.9 times more likely to die than the unvaccinated boys. The boys receiving DPT vaccine combined with OPV were 2.2 times more likely to die than the unvaccinated boys.[15]

Now why would this be? Interestingly, at least according to the study referred to above, it appears to be gender specific.

How do the vaccines affect our immune system? If we go back to what we talked about in Part One of this book, you may remember that adjuvated vaccines will activate T helper 2 (Th2) cells. The oral polio vaccine is not injected, but rather is administered the same way a person would be exposed to the natural poliovirus: via mucosal lining. Therefore, it doesn't contain adjuvants and also, it activates the T helper 1 (Th1) cells. This allows both the innate and the acquired immune system to become activated.

Morph-eus

Another concern is when we vaccinate against a germ it can adapt to its environment and survive by changing its appearance enough so the vaccine doesn't recognize it anymore. This means we now have a new germ strain created by the vaccines. Another side to this coin is the fact that usually germs already have multiple strains. Vaccinating for only one or few of them gives the other strains the opportunity to take their place.

A Dutch scientist, Dr. Frits Mooi[16], says his research suggests there is variance between the current pertussis vaccine and a new more virulent strain of the germ now in circulation.

An online article on KPBS' website discusses how people who have already been vaccinated are still contracting whooping cough. KPBS is a news media outlet provided to us by San Diego State University. The authors mention that if you were to read the package insert of "the two most common pertussis vaccines in the U.S.," you would see it says they are 85% effective.

J.D. Cherry, who was involved in the studies when the vaccines were licensed by the FDA, estimated they were 70% to 80% effective. According to the KPBS article, Dr. "Mooi said there's no way to know how effective the vaccines are because they haven't been tested against the new strain."[17]

Then there is the herd immunity concept. This is when the majority of people in a country, region or other communities are vaccinated, thereby providing a kind of protective shield for those who are not immunologically fit to receive a vaccine. On the flip side, this has also been hypothesized to alter the virus, by allowing it to adjust to the tightly packed environment.

Researchers from Finland and China used *Bordetella pertussis* to analyze how the vaccine can affect the germ.

They state:

> "[...] sequenced and analysed the complete genomes of 40 B. pertussis *strains from Finland and China, as well as 11 previously sequenced strains from the Netherlands, where different vaccination strategies have been used over the past 50 years."* [18]

In the conclusion of their study, the researchers saw:

> "[...] that evolution of the B. pertussis *population was closely associated with the country vaccination coverage."*[19]

They also noted that "the immune pressure of vaccination" dictates the evolutionary growth of *B. pertussis*.[20]

We can only imagine it's difficult enough to figure out the dangers of a vaccine covering three different illnesses, especially when also given simultaneously with other vaccines. With various countries having their own diagnostic criteria it can make it difficult for one country to know whether their results would mirror a safety trial conducted in another country. So, hypothetically could Americans, for instance, deem a vaccine safe in their country based on a trial performed in Germany?

Another concern we have is, if the criteria for what constitutes the symptoms keeps changing, should not the safety studies be reviewed or redone to mirror the updated criteria?

Chapter 27: Bias

[1] Cherry, J.D. (n.d.). *James D. Cherry, M.D.* Retrieved from www.uclahealth.org/james-cherry

[2] Krogstad, P.A. (2003). The Pediatric Infectious Diseases Society Annual Awards, 2003: Presentation of the Distinguished Physician Award to James D. Cherry, M.D. By Paul A. Krogstad, M.D. *The Pediatric Infectious Disease Journal,* 22(9), 763-764.

[3] The Embryo Project Encyclopedia. (2017, April 13). *Stanley Alan Plotkin (1932-).* Retrieved from www.embryo.asu.edu/pages/stanley-alan-plotkin-1932

[4] Cherry, J.D., Tan, T., von König, C-H., Forsyth, K.D., Thisyakorn, U., Greenberg, D., ... Plotkin, S. (2012). Clinical Definitions of Pertussis: Summary of a Global Pertussis Initiative Roundtable Meeting, February 2011. *Clinical Infectious Diseases,* 54(12), 1756-1764.

[5] Ibid.

[6] Ibid.

[7] Cherry, J.D. (2011, Deecmber 20). Why do Pertussis Vaccines Fail? [Presentation at the 9th International *Bordetella* Symposium, September 30-October 3, 2010, Baltimore, MD]. Retrieved from www.pdfs.semanticscholar.org/47ad/93234b83563f503ec4a4a1fe661bc93ee5b8.pdf

[8] Ibid.

[9] Fine, P.E.M., and Chen, R.T. (1992). Confounding in Studies of Adverse Reactions to Vaccines. *American Journal of Epidemiology,* 136(2), 121-135. Retrieved from: www.vaccinepapers.org/wp-content/uploads/confounding_in_studies_of_adverse_reactions_to_vaccines.pdf

[10] Ibid. 133.

[11] Aaby, P., Ravn, P., and Benn, C.S (2016). The WHO Review of the Possible Nonspecific Effects of Diphtheria-Tetanus-Pertussis Vaccine. *Pediatr Infect Dis J,* 35(11), 1247-1257.

Retrieved from: www.journals.lww.com/pidj/Fulltext/2016/11000/The_WHO_Review_of_the_P ossible_Nonspecific_Effects.21.aspx

[12] Mogensen, S.W., Andersen, A., Rodrigues, A., Benn, C.S., and Aaby, P. (2017). The Introduction of Diphtheria-Tetanus-Pertussis and Oral Polio Vaccine Among Young Infants in an Urban African Community: A Natural Experiment. *EBioMedicine,* 17, 192-198.

[13] Aaby, P., Benn, C., Nielsen, J., Lisse, I. M., Rodrigues, A., & Ravn, H. (2012). Testing the hypothesis that diphtheria-tetanus-pertussis vaccine has negative non-specific and sex-differential effects on child survival in high-mortality countries. *BMJ open,* 2(3), e000707. doi:10.1136/bmjopen-2011-000707

[14] Mogensen, S. W., Andersen, A., Rodrigues, A., Benn, C. S., & Aaby, P. (2017). The Introduction of Diphtheria-Tetanus-Pertussis and Oral Polio Vaccine Among Young Infants in an Urban African Community: A Natural Experiment. *EBioMedicine,* 17, 192-198.

[15] Ibid.

[16] Mooi, F.R. (n.d.). *Person: Prof. Dr. F.R. (Frits) Mooi.* Retrieved from:
www.narcis.nl/person/RecordID/PRS1242218/Language/en

[17] Faryon, J. and Crowe, K. (2010, Dec. 14th). *Immunized People Getting Whooping Cough, Experts Spar Over New Strain.* Retrieved from:
www.kpbs.org/news/2010/dec/14/immunized-people-getting-whooping-cough-experts-sp/

[18] Yinghua, X., Liu, B., Grondahl-Yli-Hannuksila, K., Tan, Y., Feng, L., Kallonen, Teemu...Zhang, S. (2015). Whole-Genome Sequencing Reveals the Effect of Vaccination on the Evolution of *Bordetella Pertussis. Scientific Reports*, 5, 12888. DOI: 10.1038/srep12888

[19] Ibid.

[20] Ibid.

CHAPTER 28

Polio—Or is it?

"When you inoculate children with a polio vaccine, you don't sleep well for two or three months."

~Jonas Salk (American medical researcher)

Polio is one of the most talked about illnesses in our modern history. The controversy surrounding this disease has become an important reference point in the development of vaccines and medicine in general. Those who lived through polio epidemics will remember the fear and the harrowing accounts of those struck down by the disease. Scientists worked around the clock to find a cure, many no doubt competing for the prestige that would come with being forever known as the one who discovered the cure for polio.

One of the vaccines released on the market ended up being contaminated and it caused quite a scare. In fact, this vaccine contamination was scarier than polio itself for some people. Some were terrified of becoming paralyzed as a result of contracting polio and couldn't wait to get their hands on a vaccine. Others were very skeptical about these vaccines, some even to the point where they questioned whether the disease was actually the result of the poliovirus.

When you think of polio, you may be thinking about one particular virus. As of today, scientists have identified three separate strains of the poliovirus. This means there are three separate germs causing polio. Therefore, in order to have complete coverage, all three germs are added to the vaccines.

The way the polioviruses affect the body ranges from no symptoms at all to paralysis or even death. The viruses enter through the mouth and some settle in the throat while others go all the way down to the intestines. These are the two areas in the body the viruses replicate and then exit with our stool and potentially infect other people.

After the viruses replicate, they reach for the blood and from there find their way to the lymph nodes and sometimes to the central nervous system.

Over half of all polio cases occur in Southeast Asia and over 20% of all cases occur in Africa and the eastern Mediterranean. In countries where polio still occurs, it's estimated that about 95% of those who contract polio don't show any major symptoms and recover without permanent damage. Nevertheless, they are carriers and can pass it along through their stools.

When doctors first started diagnosing polio, they had no way of testing each person for what was causing their symptoms. Instead, in order to diagnose a person with poliomyelitis, the doctor would perform two physicals in a 24-hour period. If the patient showed paralysis in at least one muscle group, he/she was diagnosed with polio.

Were all these documented poliomyelitis diagnoses truly caused by one of the polioviruses? We will never know.

Once they figured how to isolate the poliovirus, they were ready to develop a vaccine. In order to inactivate the virus, they used formaldehyde. Unfortunately, there were problems where the virus came back to life in the vaccines. So instead of vaccinating those with a weakened virus, they injected full blown poliovirus into people. This caused more cases of poliolytic paralysis.

When vaccines came out, coincidentally or not, the way polio was diagnosed also changed. Instead of diagnosis being dependent on the symptoms occurring in two examinations within a 24-hour period, it was two examinations within a 60-day period. Most people recovered from the paralysis before the 60-day period was over. People who would previously have been diagnosed with polio were no longer diagnosed with polio.

Mix and match

We studied polio statistics before and after the final changes on polio diagnosis, which was in 1960. Aseptic meningitis used to be diagnosed as nonparalytic poliomyelitis.

One paper explains the three main categories of poliomyelitis as follows:

> *"These have been categorized into inapparent infection without symptoms, mild illness (abortive poliomyelitis), aseptic meningitis (nonparalytic poliomyelitis), and paralytic poliomyelitis."*[1]

Polio statistics are normally divided into categories showing how severe the polio cases were with a column of total polio cases at the end. We looked only at the numbers of total polio cases[23] rather than per severity.

Another point to mention before we present our graph (see Chart 1), a child neurology textbook[4], lists viruses with similar symptoms to polio. These include viruses such as Adenovirus, Coxsackieviruses (AKA atypical polio), Echo virus, and Roseola. Before polio was identified by symptoms, these viruses were sometimes diagnosed as polio.

For this book, however, we have chosen to stick to aseptic meningitis due to unreliable margin of error, as we were unable to find a website with accurate data for us to graph the other viruses. We just wanted to see if there was a trend and whether even just one diagnostic adjustment would change the graph by using the incidence rates in the US referenced to above.

We noticed an upward trend in aseptic anemia as the polio cases declined. Even before aseptic meningitis, it appears polio cases had plummeted. We cannot help but wonder what the true trend looks like with all the diagnostic adjustments considered.

In 1959, scientists looked into a polio incident that occurred in the Detroit, Michigan area, the previous year when 867 individuals were diagnosed with polio (520 paralytic and 347 nonparalytic). Staff at Herman Kiefer Hospital in Detroit, Michigan, collected stool samples from 556 of its polio-diagnosed patients for testing.[5]

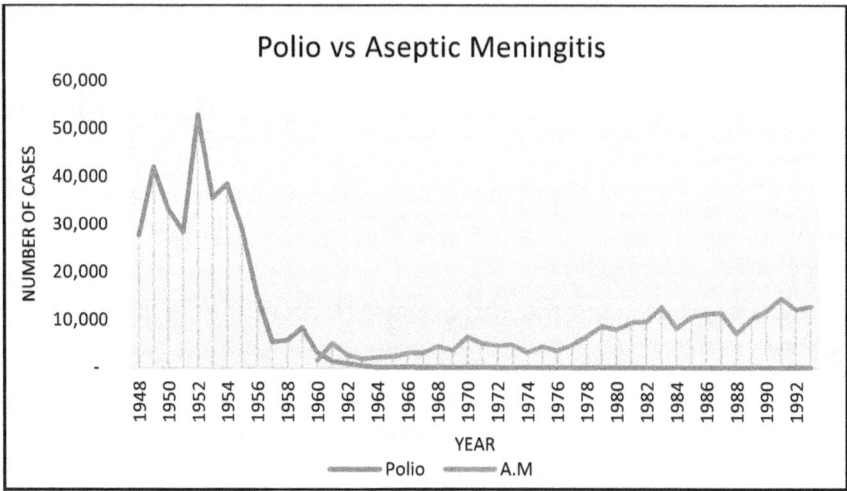

Chart 1

Some 225 patients whose stool samples were submitted for testing were diagnosed with paralytic poliomyelitis and 208 with nonparalytic poliomyelitis[6]. As you may recall, there are three types of polio: Type 1, 2 and 3. All three types were tested in the patients, but only type one and three were detected.

Their findings in the stool samples from patients with paralytic polio found 162 of them were positive for type 1 or 3. They also tested the samples for Coxsackievirus and ECHO, but the 63 remaining patients tested negative for any of the viruses. This means that out of the 225 patients diagnosed with paralytic polio, only 162 or 72% of them actually had confirmed test results for a poliovirus.[7]

In the nonparalytic group, this was a little more interesting. Out of the 208 patients, only 42 of them tested positive for poliovirus type 1 or 3. Another 44 patients tested positive for coxsackie and ECHO viruses, while the remaining 185 tested negative for any of the viruses. This means that only 20% of the patients had diagnosable poliomyelitis.[8]

If these types of errors in the pre-vaccination statistics were taken into account, we can't help but wonder whether the earlier epidemics were actually caused by polio or something else. Meaning, did the pre-vaccination period really consist of that many cases of polio?

Another interesting factor is that around the same time, the diagnosis was not the only thing that changed. The definition of what constitutes an epidemic changed as well. Instead of it being 20 polio cases in a population of 100,000, it was now 35 polio cases in a population of 100,000.[9] The requirement almost doubled. It must have been quite difficult to spark an epidemic when not only were more sick people required to constitute an epidemic, but the diagnosis was changed drastically. There just weren't enough individuals left sick with the actual virus.

There are many arguments over how all these requirements and criteria were introduced in order to make the vaccine appear safer. We feel there is another factor that should not be underestimated, and that is once they began working on a vaccine and identifying the virus in laboratories, scientists learned more about viruses and its behavior and that of other viruses as well.

So, this appears to us to be a natural evolution—a redefinition of the disease. But that doesn't explain why this wasn't considered when the statistics or case studies were being publicized.

It's alive

Angela Matysiak wrote an article in *MIT Technology Review* where she noted that Salk's vaccine was not a great success:

> *"One of the main concerns was that the Salk vaccine did not prevent infection in the gut and thus did not break the chain of transmission."*[10]

Many of you may have heard of the "Cutter incidence." When Jonas Salk introduced the very first polio vaccine, it was produced by Cutter Laboratories. As with so many other vaccines, the developers used formalin to kill the virus. When using a chemical to kill a virus, it's important to use just the right amount of chemical. With the polio vaccine the objective was to inactivate or kill the virus so it wouldn't make you sick.

In his book *The Cutter Incident,* Dr. Paul Offit shares the tragic story about scientists with Cutter Laboratories mass producing Salk's vaccine and how in 1955 about 400,000 individuals, of whom the majority of were children, were vaccinated with it. After being vaccinated, recipients contracted polio. In fact, 40,000 became sick, leaving 200 children "severely paralyzed" and 10 died.[11]

Dr. Paul Offit writes:

> *"Children given Cutter's vaccine were more likely to be paralyzed in their arms, more likely to suffer severe and permanent paralysis, more likely to require breathing assistance in iron lungs, and more likely die than did children naturally infected with polio."*[12]

Below is a picture you may recognize. It has infamously been associated with the scare of The Cutter incident. (One tiny little detail to keep in mind: The Cutter Incident occurred in 1955). According to Smithsonian National Museum of American History, this picture is a staged scene in the gym at Rancho Los Amigos National Rehabilitation Center.[13] According to the Polio Survivors Association, this picture "was taken in 1953 as part of an information film produced by the March of Dimes."[14]

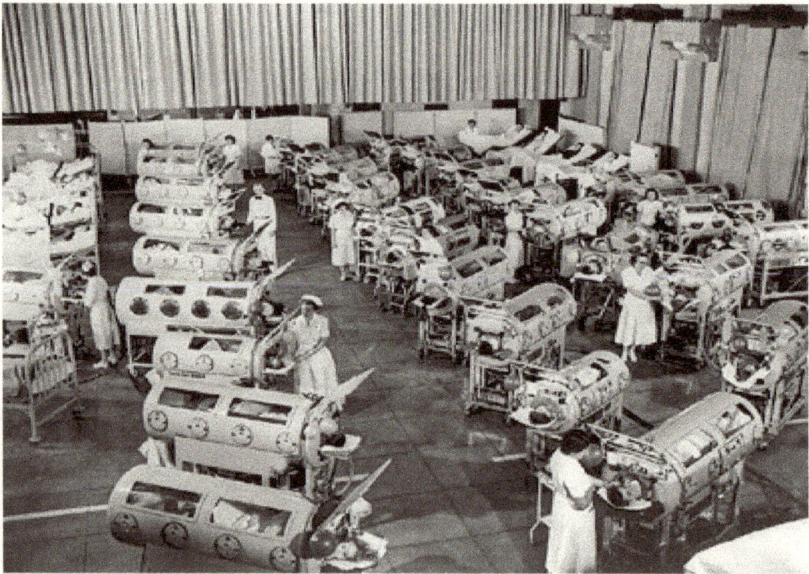

The Smithsonian website underneath the picture states:

> *"At first glance, this image shocks and saddens from the enormity of the problem of sick children in need of iron lungs. On closer examination, it is clear that the equipment that usually accompanied people using iron lungs, such as tracheotomy tubes and pumps and tankside tables, is not present [...]."*[15]

Wikipedia states the picture is a "Photo of polio patients in iron lungs during 1953 epidemic," but this description is sourced to a book that appears to believe the photo is from an epidemic in 1952:

> *"1952, the worst epidemic year in history: polio patients in iron lungs and rocking beds at Rancho Los Amigos Medical Center, Downey, California."*[16]

Regardless of the discrepancy, we feel certain the picture was taken prior to the Cutter incident.

There were other companies besides Cutter Laboratories that produced the disease-causing Salk vaccines, but none were stigmatized like Cutter Laboratories was. This makes us wonder how many individuals actually became sick from polio vaccines. Keep in mind this happened at the same time as polio incidences dropped and the incidences of other illnesses rose. Which begs the question whether it's possible a mutated polio vaccine-strain could have played a hand in this rise in polio-like illnesses. Early in 1960, they started using Sabin's oral polio vaccine instead.

Chapter 28: Polio – Or is it?

[1] Mehndiratta, M. M., Mehndiratta, P., & Pande, R. (2014). Poliomyelitis: historical facts, epidemiology, and current challenges in eradication. *The Neurohospitalist*, 4(4), 223-229.

[2] The College of Physicians of Philadelphia. (2018). *U.S. Polio Cases 1952-1962*. Retrieved from www.historyofvaccines.org/content/us-polio-cases-1952-1962

[3] Post-Polio Health International. (n.d.). *Incidence Rates of Poliomyelitis in US*. Retrieved from www.post-polio.org/ir-usa.html

[4] Menkes, J.H. and Sarnat, H.B. (Eds.). (2000). *Child Neurology* (6th ed., pp. 522-526). Philadelphia, PA: Lippincott Williams & Wilkins.

[5] MOLNER, J. G., & AGATE, G. H. (1960). Final report of poliomyelitis epidemic in Detroit and Wayne County, 1958. *Public health reports (Washington, D.C. : 1896)*, 75(11), 1031-1043.

[6] Ibid.

[7] Ibid.

[8] Ibid.

[9] Ratner, H., Cox, H.R., Greenberg, B.G, Kleinman, H., and Meier, P. (1960). "The Present Status of Polio Vaccines." *Illinois Medical Journal*, 118(2), 19

[10] Matysiak, A. (2005, Jul 1st.). *The Myth of Jonas Salk*. Retrieved from www.technologyreview.com/s/404390/the-myth-of-jonas-salk/

[11] Offit, P. (2005) *The Cutter Incident: How America's First Polio Vaccine Led to the Growing Vaccine Crisis* (1st ed.). U.S: Yale University Press.

[12] Ibid. p.86

[13] Smithsonian National Museum of American History. (n.d.). *Understanding Historical Photos*. Retrieved from www.amhistory.si.edu/polio/historicalphotos/index.htm

[14] Polio Survivors Association. (2018). *Pictures of Polio*. Retrieved from www.polioassociation.org/pictures.html

[15] Smithsonian National Museum of American History. (n.d.). *Understanding Historical Photos*. Retrieved from www.amhistory.si.edu/polio/historicalphotos/index.htm

[16] Smith, J.S. (1990). *Patenting the sun: polio and the Salk vaccine* (1st ed.). New York, NY: W. Morrow

CHAPTER 29

Polio—Syndromes

*"…Your body is SET to repair and restore,
not degenerate."*

~Dr. Jack Stockwell CGP

Chronic Fatigue Syndrome (CFS), also known as Myalgic Encephalomyelitis (ME) or ME/CFS, is one serious illness that has been linked to polio.

It has been estimated that "15–30 million people around the world are suffering from ME"[1]. Some argue this new syndrome has aided in the eradication of polio. Meaning, because the vaccines have caused mutations in the polioviruses, this syndrome is actually a form of polio. Therefore, it appears the diagnosis has changed yet again.

Would we still have a polio epidemic or scare today had the definition never changed?

It's also argued that ME/CFS includes what used to be called Atypical Polio or coxsackievirus. (As you may recall from the study in Michigan, many of the polio patients tested positive for the coxsackievirus and not polioviruses). We did some digging into this assumption to see where the association would be. Some people who became ill with a viral infection, including the coxsackievirus, came down with post-viral fatigue syndrome (PVFS) which is sometimes written as postviral fatigue syndrome (PFS).

Authors of an article from 1988 conclude:

> *"However, it is likely that although enteroviruses are major aetiological agents of PFS, other viruses, particularly Epstein-Barr virus, may induce the syndrome. We suggest that this disease is a chronic metabolic myopathy induced by persistent virus infection."*[2]

What is PVFS? The first thing we did was to look it up in ICD-11, the most recent ICD code we could find, to see if it's a recognized disease. We found it under the code 8E49. According to that code, this syndrome includes benign myalgic encephalomyelitis and chronic fatigue syndrome.[3] We understand that to be the same as ME/CFS.

The encyclopedia for ME lists multiple studies where mice infected with the coxsackievirus showed that exercise had detrimental effects on their health. It continues on to say that one of its symptoms is induced aseptic meningitis (nonparalytic polio) and that it has "been linked to myalgic encephalomyelitis and chronic fatigue syndrome, fibromyalgia, as well as type 1 diabetes."[4]

According the *Oxford Textbook of Medicine:*

> *"Chronic fatigue syndrome (CFS) is also known as post-viral fatigue syndrome, neurasthenia, and myalgic encephalomyelitis. All describe an idiopathic syndrome characterized by disabling fatigue and other symptoms occurring chronically and exacerbated by minimal exertion."*[5]

We feel we have a good enough reason to consider ME/CFS to be identical to ME/CFS/PVFS.

You'd expect there to be differences in diseases caused by different viruses, but if these viruses are all of the same family then perhaps it's not surprising there are similarities.

We found a paper written by, among others, Dr. R. Bruno[6], former director of the Post-Polio Institute and current director of International Center for Post-Polio Education and Research.

After explaining there are other types of viral infections on the brain, the authors state:

> *"Still other agents (e.g., Coxsackie, echo and herpes viruses) have been associated with symptoms of chronic fatigue. And, although there is no convincing clinical or immunological evidence that post-polio fatigue or CFS is caused by a persistent poliovirus infection, only poliovirus has been directly or indirectly associated so often throughout this century with acute and chronic impairment of cortical activation, decreased attention and symptoms of fatigue."*[7]

216

But if ME/CFS is a type of polio, why doesn't everyone exposed to the relevant viruses develop ME/CFS just as they did in the case of polio?

Numbers and figures

The CDC appears to have recently changed its breakdown of the symptoms for contracting polio. It's surprising to us they don't acknowledge it or even mention that in the past year some new research has come to light that has drastically changed the percentages.

In 2017 their webpage stated that 95% of those infected with polio had no visible symptoms[8]. In 2018 this percentage dropped to show 72% of those infected had no visible symptoms[9].

We will stick to the most recent figures. In addition to the 72% having no visible symptoms, they state that 25% will have flu-like symptoms that go away in only a few days. These cases combined mean 97% of those with poliovirus will probably never know they were affected. This leaves only 3% of those infected with poliovirus to have serious symptoms as opposed to less than 1% as specified on their webpage in 2017. Both statistical versions agree that 10% or less out of those who become paralyzed die.

By using the CDC's most recent statistics, let's see if we can put this into a perspective. Say 1,000,000 people become infected with polio. Some 720,000 of them have no clue they are harboring the virus at all. Another 250,000 feel like they may have the flu. They may have a sore throat, a headache or feel tired, but in a few days the symptoms are gone and they most likely never knew it was polio. This adds up to 970,000 individuals with either no symptoms or minor symptoms. This leaves 30,000 individuals who will react much stronger to the poliovirus. Some 200 individuals will experience paralysis or weakening of limbs, and between four and 20 individuals will die.

Normally when there is an outbreak of a disease, it doesn't affect as many as 1,000,000 individuals. If 100 people contracted polio, the media would be all over it with sensational headlines announcing the return of the deadly paralyzing virus. How deadly or paralyzing would it really be if a 100 people became infected? Statistically, 97 of them would never even know they had polio until they were tested for it. If the stats are correct, the disease would also leave their body without much, if any, medical attention. Which begs the question how accurate such statistics are.

Another page on CDC's website refers to nonparalytic aseptic meningitis and flaccid paralysis as clinical features of polio.[10] We've come to realize that it's an entire project on its own just to map out the diagnostical changes to solve the polio conundrum.

China's polio

Since we are on the path of neurological diseases, why don't we throw Guillain-Barré Syndrome (GBS) into the mix? This disease has been tied to multiple vaccines, including polio vaccine. We won't discuss it further in this chapter, but we want to share with you our discovery of a syndrome we had never heard of until now, Chinese Paralytic Syndrome (CPS).

In a thesis on the subject, written for *partial fulfillment of requirements for the degree of Master of Science,* the student explains simply that:

> "CPS is often confused with GBS. From a clinical perspective, the only differences between the CPS and GBS stems from the fact that CPS has a seasonal variation and is predominantly seen in northern China. It has been suggested that CPS is not a variant of GBS but a variant of poliomyelitis caused by an altered poliovirus."[11]

Apart from that, it appears new names for neurological diseases are constantly increasing. Soon, the neurological effects of vaccines will disappear into oblivion because the categories are too many to singularly show a statistical significance worthy of inclusion in reports.

Africa's polio

A cheaper version of the polio vaccine is the live oral polio vaccine. The danger with using a live viral vaccine is the high likelihood of the virus mutating. Sometimes the mutations can be even more dangerous than the strain it's derived from. As mentioned earlier, polioviruses are passed on via feces. This can be especially troubling in countries such as Nigeria where the water source is used for multiple purposes like bathing and drinking. The oral version is used in Nigeria and in 2007 nearly 70 children became paralyzed from a mutated poliovirus traced back to the vaccine.

An online CBS news article from 2009 reports that Nigerian leaders and residents have been skeptical about vaccines for quite some time. Back in 2003, rumors had it that the polio vaccine was laced with sterilizing agents and HIV. The Nigerian authorities put a stop to all polio vaccinations. Tests were performed to ensure there were no such contaminants or tampering with the vaccines. In 2004, when these were shown to be empty rumors, the Nigerian authorities continued vaccinating its people.

Besides Nigeria, polio persists in a few other countries, including Afghanistan, Angola, Chad, China, Egypt, Haiti, India, Madagascar, Pakistan, Philippines and Sudan. The polio strains causing illnesses in these countries can often be traced back to vaccine-derived polioviruses (VDPVs).

A paper published in 2005 highlights the struggles of eradicating polio and how the use of oral polio vaccine is making eradication more difficult. The authors discuss the advantages of injectable polio vaccines (IPV) by summarizing another study from the same year, co-authored by Plotkin[12]:

> *"[...] demonstrate that enhanced-potency inactivated vaccine reduces both the titer of poliovirus excreted in stools and the duration of excretion. These findings suggest that currently available IPV will inhibit circulation of polioviruses and, consequently, should provide a greater degree of herd immunity than the original Salk vaccine."*[13]

The authors concern is the consistent use of the oral polio vaccine (OPV) in countries where the vaccine coverage is not high enough to cause herd-immunity.

They state:

> *"Many of the poorest countries in the world are unable to vaccinate even 50% of their children. Under these circumstances, continuing to use OPV after eradication is very risky."*[14]

This fear makes sense considering how easily the live virus in the oral vaccine is spread via feces, thereby giving more opportunity for revertant[15] strains to cause vaccine-associated paralytic poliomyelitis to occur.

The comment in the paper co-authored by Plotkin, regarding areas that are unvaccinated, would be of concern in countries where less than half the children are vaccinated.

They explain:

> *"[...] the spread of excreted vaccine-derived strains would be much higher and could result in their own transformation into pathogenic variants. This provides additional justification for the continued use of IPV, at least until the risk of reemergence of poliovirus is eliminated."*[16]

The concerns scientists have with polioviruses and their mutations may already be too late to resolve the way they hoped. When children aren't being vaccinated, as is the case in Africa, mutations from the vaccines may already be out of scientists' control.

The fear Nigerians have of the vaccines had much to do with the above-mentioned rumor of the vaccines being "deliberately contaminated with anti-fertility agents and the HIV virus." [17] Some reports add "cancerous agents" to the list of concerns.[18] As a result many Nigerians were too afraid to get vaccinated against polio. Consequently, it's believed that 789 individuals became infected with polio in 2004.[19] As far as we know, there has never been any official evidence the vaccines were deliberately contaminated with any of these agents. Western nations have seldom been honest and upfront with the African people, so we can see how such rumors can cause vaccine paranoia.

Chapter 29: Polio – Syndromes
[1] ME Action. (2018). *What is ME*. Retrieved from www.meaction.net/about/what-is-me/
[2] Archard, L. C., Bowles, N. E., Behan, P. O., Bell, E. J., & Doyle, D. (1988). Postviral fatigue syndrome: persistence of enterovirus RNA in muscle and elevated creatine kinase. *Journal of the Royal Society of Medicine*, 81(6), 326-329.
[3] The World Health Organization. (2018). *ICD-11 for Mortality and Morbidity Statistics (2018).* Retrieved from www.icd.who.int/browse11/l-m/en#/http://id.who.int/icd/entity/569175314

[4] ME Action (2018, Nov. 6th). *Coxsackie B virus*. Retrieved from www.me-pedia.org/wiki/Coxsackie_B_virus
[5] Oxford Medicine Online. (2018). *Oxford Textbook of Medicine*. Retrieved from www.oxfordmedicine.com/view/10.1093/med/9780199204854.001.1/med-9780199204854-chapter-260504
[6] Post Polio Info. (n.d.). *Welcome to the International Centre for Polio*. Retrieved from www.postpolioinfo.com/bruno.php
[7] Bruno, R.L, Frick, N.M, Creange, S., Zimmerman, R., & Lewis, T. (1996). Polioencephalitis and the Brain Fatigue Generator Model of Post-Viral Fatigue Syndromes. *Journal of Chronic Fatigue Syndrome*, 2(2-3), 5-27
[8] The Center for Disease Control and Prevention. (2011). *Vaccines and Preventable Diseases:*
Polio Disease In-Short. Retrieved from web.archive.org/web/20130713110546/http:/www.cdc.gov/vaccines/vpd-vac/polio/in-short-both.htm
[9] Center for Disease Control and Prevention. (2017, July 25). *What is Polio?* Retrieved from www.cdc.gov/polio/about/
[10] Center for Disease Control and Prevention. (2015, September 29). *Epidemiology and Prevention of Vaccine-Preventable Diseases*. Retrieved from www.cdc.gov/vaccines/pubs/pinkbook/polio.html
[11] Allen, K.J. (2000) *Construction and Application of flaA Sigma-28 Promoter Fusions to the Virulence and Ecology of Campylobacter Jejuni*. (Master of Science Thesis, University of Guelph, Ontario, Canada). Retrieved from www.collectionscanada.gc.ca/obj/s4/f2/dsk3/ftp04/MQ56299.pdf
[12] Laassri, M, Lottenbach, K., Belshe, R., Wolff, M., Rennels, M., Plotkin, S., and Churnakov, K. (2005). Effect of different vaccination schedules on excretion of oral poliovirus vaccine strains. *J Infect Dis*, 192(12), 2092-2098.
[13] Hull, H.F and Minor, P.D. (2005). "When Can We Stop Using Oral Poliovirus Vaccine?" *The Journal of Infectious Diseases*, 192(12), 2033–2035, www.doi.org/10.1086/498171
[14] Ibid.
[15] "a mutant gene, individual, or strain that regains a former capability (such as the production of a particular protein) by undergoing further mutation" www.merriam-webster.com/dictionary/revertant

[16] Laassri, M, Lottenbach, K., Belshe, R., Wolff, M., Rennels, M., Plotkin, S., and Churnakov, K. (2005). Effect of different vaccination schedules on excretion of oral poliovirus vaccine strains. *J Infect Dis*, 192(12), 2092-2098.

[17] Yahya, M. (2007). Polio vaccines—"no thank you!" barriers to polio eradication in Northern Nigeria. *African Affairs, 106(423), 185-204*

[18] Jegede A. S. (2007). What led to the Nigerian boycott of the polio vaccination campaign?. *PLoS medicine*, 4(3), e73.

[19] Nature. (2018) *Polio: Eradication.* Retrieved from www.nature.com/nature/focus/polio/eradication.html

CHAPTER 30

SV40 scare

*"Stuff that's hidden and murky and
ambiguous is scary because you don't know what
it does."*

~Jerry Garcia (American musician)

The National Vaccine Information Center (NVIC) posted a statement
given at *FDA Vaccines & Related Biological Products Advisory Committee
Meeting May 7, 2010* advising:

> *"A 1973 prospective study of more than 50,000
> pregnancies concluded that inactivated polio vaccines
> given to pregnant women in that study between 1959 and
> 1965 were associated with excess malignancies and brain
> tumors in children born to those mothers."*[1]

We couldn't find a source for this study, so we were unable to read it
ourselves. Instead, we searched for studies that researched that exact
topic. The two most recent scientific discussions we found on this exact
topic was a paper published in 2004 and a book on mesothelioma
(tumors). Both of these would have been available at the time of the
committee meeting.

The authors of the 2004 paper:

> *"[...] studied, 54,796 children enrolled in the US-based
> Collaborative Perinatal Project (CPP) in 1959–1966, 52 of
> whom developed cancer by their eighth birthday."*[2]

They conclude their study by explaining they:

> *"[...] found no consistent relation between maternal SV40
> seroconversion during pregnancy and cancer in children."*[3]

Then two years later, in 2006 in a book on mesothelioma tumors, we found a section written about this very subject. The book, which is not about vaccines, states how multiple studies came to the conclusion there's no association between SV-40 and cancer. The authors point out there are other studies that have shown an association.

Their conclusion was that:

> *"[...] it is currently not possible to establish SV40-positive and SV40-negative cohorts that are large enough for a statistically significant study."*[4]

Instead, the authors suggest that:

> *"Because the development of most cancers is multifactorial, it is likely that SV40 acts with other agents or factors to cause mesothelioma."*[5]

Due to the complexities of finding subjects that can give researchers a reliable outcome, we steered away from these types of studies and looked into animal studies. We are fully aware of the biological differences in species, but nonetheless, this is what scientists have to work with.

In the above-mentioned book, the editors do exactly that: they give more confidence to the results of animal studies. They state that when newborn animals are injected with SV40, it triggers the development of various tumors. In order to receive the same result in adult animals, a much higher dose of SV40 was needed. The authors argue this could have something to do with the developing immune system:

> *"The increased sensitivity of newborn animals to SV40-induced tumorigenesis may be a result of their more immature immune systems. Immunosuppression may also make humans more susceptible to the carcinogenic effects of SV40."*[6]

This is how the authors explain how asbestos and SV40, together, trigger the formation of tumor cells. They state:

> *"The possibility that SV40 and asbestos may also act as co-carcinogens in vivo is important, since SV40 is frequently found in mesothelioma patients with a history of asbestos exposure."*[7]

Not that we know much about the history of asbestos, but we are guessing there is some legitimate dot-connecting between asbestos and cancer. Anything that weakens the cell will allow germs easier access to, or perhaps even facilitate an ambush on, our immune system.

Not quite dead yet

All polio vaccines produced in the US in the period 1954 through 1960 were infected with the Simian Virus 40 (SV40). This DNA virus has the ability to cause cancer in hamsters by splicing its DNA with DNA in the tumor cells. Its DNA did not appear to splice with human DNA, so the question was whether it would cause cancer in humans.[8]

The authors of that study explain that viral DNA which does not become a part of the human DNA will replicate a thousand-fold and kill the human cells.

There are incidences where formaldehyde has been a problem. It turns out that the amount of formaldehyde it takes to inactivate the polioviruses is not necessarily enough to kill the SV40 virus. But this was not the case in this this instance.

The authors explain:

> *"We determined that the procedure used by this manufacturer to inactivate SV40 in oral poliovirus vaccine seed stocks based on heat inactivation in the presence of $MgCl_2$ did not completely inactivate SV40."*[9]

$MgCl_2$ is Magnesium Chloride and we didn't find it on the CDC's list of vaccine ingredients.[10]

The authors continue:

> *"These SV40-contaminated vaccines were produced from early 1960s to about 1978 and were used throughout the world. [...] and emphasize the importance of using well-characterized cell substrates that are free from adventitious agents. Moreover, our results indicate possible geographic differences in SV40 exposure and offer*

*a possible explanation for the different percentage of SV40-
positive tumors detected in some laboratories."*[11]

It's now widely known and accepted as fact that some polio vaccines
were contaminated by a rhesus monkey virus called simian virus 40
(SV40), which is a DNA tumor virus.[12] By 1961, all vaccines were
assumed to be free of the SV40 virus. In order to make sure this was the
case, the WHO tested laboratories in 13 different countries for SV40
contamination. They all came out free from SV40 contamination except
for the eastern European vaccine manufacturer (EEVM). It so happens
that this laboratory distributed these vaccines all around the world. The
last contaminated batch was produced in 1978.[13]

As mentioned above, some argue this virus is the cause of cancers.
Although likely, research on this hypothesis has not, as far as we could
determine, been overly convincing. We came across one paper where the
authors looked at 13 separate studies on the matter.

They conclude:

> *"SV40 is associated significantly with brain tumors, bone
> cancers, malignant mesothelioma, and non-Hodgkin's
> lymphoma."*[14]

It seems we are so intent on eradicating the poliovirus we are too blind
to see the effects it has already had on sufferers. Instead of focusing on
polio, we should probably focus on the various viruses and toxins that
cause paralysis. There are other viruses that can cause paralysis that we
don't even talk about. And do we really know if kids in these Third World
countries are experiencing paralysis because of polio or something else?

Time, effort, money and publicity can stand in the way of recognizing
the most logical solutions. As mentioned earlier in this book: sometimes
the foundation of stronger health is as simple as the washing of hands.[15]

Chapter 30: SV40 scare

[1] National Vaccine Information Center (NVIC). (n.d.). *NVIC Statement on Finding of PCV DNA Sequences in Rotavirus Vaccines.* Retrieved from www.nvic.org/Downloads/barbara-loe-fisher-statement-may-7-2010.aspx

[2] Engels, E.A., Chen, J., Viscidi, R.D., Shah, K.V., Daniel, R.W., Chatterjee, N., and Klebanoff, M.A. (2004). Poliovirus Vaccination during Pregnancy, Maternal Seroconversion to Simian Virus 40, and Risk of Childhood Cancer. *Am J Epidemiol,* 160(4). DOI: 10.1093/aje/kwh219

[3] Ibid.

[4] Powers, A., Bocchetta, M., and Carbone, M. (2006). Viral factors in the pathogenesis of malignant mesothelioma. O'Byrne, K., and Rusch, V. (Eds.). *Malignant Pleural Mesothelioma* (1st ed., pp. 147-162). New York: Oxford University Press.

[5] Ibid

[6] Ibid.

[7] Ibid.

[8] Cutrone, R., Lednicky, J., Dunn, G., Rizzo, P., Bocchetta, M., Chumakov, K. … Carbone, M. (2005). Some oral poliovirus vaccines were contaminated with infectious SV40 after 1961. *Cancer* Res, 65(22), 10273-10279.

[9] Ibid.

[10] The Center of Disease Control and Prevention. (2012). *Vaccine Excipient & Media Summary*
Retrieved from
www.cdc.gov/vaccines/pubs/pinkbook/downloads/appendices/B/excipient-table-2.pdf

[11] Cutrone, R., Lednicky, J., Dunn, G., Rizzo, P., Bocchetta, M., Chumakov, K. … Carbone, M. (2005). Some oral poliovirus vaccines were contaminated with infectious SV40 after 1961. *Cancer* Res, 65(22), 10273-10279.

[12] Corallini, A., Mazzoni, E., Taronna, A., Manfrini, M., Carandina, G. Guerra, G. … Tognon, M.G. (2012) Specific antibodies reacting with simian virus 40 capsid protein mimotopes in serum samples from healthy blood donors. *Human Immunology*, 73(5), 502-510 www.doi.org/10.1016/j.humimm.2012.02.009

[13] Cutrone, R., Lednicky, J., Dunn, G., Rizzo, P., Bocchetta, M., Chumakov, K. … Carbone, M. (2005). Some oral poliovirus vaccines were contaminated with infectious SV40 after 1961. *Cancer* Res, 65(22), 10273-10279.

[14] Vilchez, R.A, Kozinetz, C.A, Arringtom, A.S, Madden, C.R., and Butel, J.S. (2003) Simian virus 40 in human cancers. *Am J Med*, 114(8) , 675 - 684

[15] Wikipedia. (2018, December 3). *Ignaz Semmelweis.* Retrieved from www.en.wikipedia.org/wiki/Ignaz_Semmelweis

Polio—The controversy continues

"In vaccines, from those people who work at the most local level to those people who develop, who invent, who create vaccines, we all have the power to change the world."

~Dr. Andrew Wakefield.

What appears to be happening around the world is that the three polio strains used in vaccines are making way for other polio-like viruses to take the place of polio. When we alter the population's immune response to cater for specific strains, we're not just altering our body's reaction, but also our environmental balance of opportunistic infections. We are therefore not surprised to see such syndromes as ME/CFS and GBS on the rise.

When less than one percent of children who contract polio become paralyzed, why does it seem that so many children have ended up paralyzed after being vaccinated for polio? Even if we include other enteroviruses, which seem to increase in number each time we look them up, we can't help but wonder was the fearmongering based on media hype or was paralysis truly an adverse reaction (in children) to being vaccinated?

It's poison

The answer to this question would, in our opinion, be largely hypothetical.

Could there possibly be something to the DDT theory?

Dichlorodiphenyltrichloroethane, or DDT, is a toxin believed to have similar effects on our system as vaccine ingredients are thought to have. Some even believe it is the true cause of the polio-associated paralysis. If we consider this theory for a moment, perhaps the intense DDT spraying children were subjected to in the decade 1943–1952, may have wreaked havoc on our immune systems and allowed the viruses to affect them in ways it would never have naturally occurred. Similar to asbestos perhaps?

In 1939, the Swiss chemist, Paul Hermann Müller,[1] when searching for a toxin that would harm insects without affecting mammals (i.e. humans), discovered the power of DDT to fight "diseases transmittable by insects, diseases such as typhus, malaria and sandfly fever." This earned him the Nobel Prize in 1948.[2]

Dr. Müller was hired by the Swiss company J. R. Geigy AG where he made this discovery and together with Geigy holds the patent on DDT. Later on, J.R. Geigy AG became one of the companies to merge into the pharmaceutical company Novartis.

Did Dr. Müller underestimate the harmful effects of DDT?

We know there wasn't much DDT sprayed into the environment before 1943. It didn't really enter the US until after WW2, but by then it had been a great success in Europe, especially Italy, keeping malaria incidences down. After observing the great success using DDT for malaria control, Merck got in the forefront introducing DDT to the US.

Author Jim West[3] has shown an interesting correlation between DDT production and polio. In a response to an article published in the *British Medical Journal,* West gives examples of why he feels DDT is bad. One such example is in the beginning of 1950s, bodies of calves displaying signs of paralysis and high levels of DDT were discovered in the US and Switzerland.[4]

What those who lived through it may know perhaps is that it was most generously applied in 1951–1952 at the end of the so-called DDT decade. If we look at our polio chart from a couple of chapters ago, we can see that in 1952 polio statistics flared up.

In 1953, in what was surely purely coincidental, Dr. Kumm,[5] a DDT proponent, became the new head of polio research at the National Foundation for Infantile Paralysis (NFIP).[6] As the link referenced above shows, he was heavily involved in malaria research around the world, which included the use of DDT.

One would think if anyone was qualified to recognize a connection between DDT and neurological damage, Dr. Kumm would be high on that list.

In 1954, the injectable polio vaccine was developed by Dr. Salk, licensed and then withdrawn. In the meantime, polio cases continued to drop. In 1956, organo-phosphates replaced the later prohibited DDT. From 1957, when the polio epidemic had almost ended, the injectable vaccine was revised and used for the first time for mass vaccination.

Hybrids

In Germany, where the vaccine was reintroduced, deaths not only increased, but nearly doubled. The injectable polio replaced Sabin's oral polio vaccine. There was an extreme drop in polio-related deaths in 1962. Interestingly, this was at the same period when less children were being vaccinated and the vaccine did not cover all three viruses.

One possible explanation for the decline is before 1962 the most common form of polio was non-paralytic polio (aseptic meningitis). Its main symptoms (muscle cramps, but no paralysis) are virtually identical to meningitis and encephalitis, which results in inflammation of the brain membranes.

Africa has struggled with polio far more than any other part of the world. In 2015, there were 26,052 cases of acute flaccid paralysis (AFP) reported in 47 African countries. Interestingly enough, the same report showed zero cases of wild polio infections and 18 vaccine strain polio infections.[7]

In addition, the report also listed researchers' results from stool samples from people diagnosed with AFP in the WHO region from 2015 and 2016. Out of the six WHO regions (Africa, Americas, Eastern Mediterranean, European, South-East Asia and Western Pacific), only one region found wild poliovirus in the stool samples. In 2015, in the Eastern Mediterranean 25,827 samples were collected of which 74 were wild and 951 originated from the Sabin vaccine. In 2016, they collected 31,928 samples of which 33 were wild and 1,612 were from the Sabin vaccine.

Every single WHO region found Sabin polio strain in some of the AFP patients' stool samples. In 2015, in all WHO regions combined, researchers tested 192,250 stool samples from AFP patients. Out of these, only 74 were from wild polio strain and 8,209 samples from Sabin's vaccine strain. In 2016, they tested 220,920 stool samples. They found 37 wild polio strains and 11,972 Sabin strains. It appears that while wild polio is decreasing, vaccine-derived polio appears to be on the rise.[8]

Before the AFP diagnosis was set in motion, if most of those cases were considered polio then surely that in itself would have made polio appear rampant and widespread, or epidemic if you prefer.

Recently in the US, the CDC in Atlanta reported a surge of the polio-like condition, acute flaccid myelitis (AFM). In late October 2018, the CDC posted on their website that this condition:

> *"[...] affects the nervous system, specifically the area of spinal cord called gray matter, which causes the muscles and reflexes in the body to become weak. [...]. Still, CDC estimates that less than one in a million people in the United States will get AFM every year."[9]*

The following are listed as possible causes of this condition: poliovirus, non-polio enterovirus, West Nile virus (WNV) and adenoviruses. Interestingly, the Washington State Health Department link refers to AFM as being the same as poliomyelitis. They go through all the criteria for both and in some places they even refer to the condition as "AFM/Polio"[10].

By now you may be wondering how AFM differs from AFP. The same link as the Washington State Health Department link we referenced above explains that AFM is a subset of AFP, the main difference being that AFM includes abnormalities in the grey matter or CSF pleocytosis. On their link, they have added an informative figure that explains the differences very clearly.[11]

When we looked up confirmed cases of AFM on the CDC's website in October, 2018, it showed 80 cases. By December 12 that same year, when we revisited the same page, the confirmed cases were up to 158[12] individuals diagnosed with AFM. The CDC is hard at work investigating other patients. It will be interesting to follow the course of development and identification of AFM.

Virus wants to stay

In May 2010, there was a mass Oral polio vaccine (OPV) campaign in Mexico. Researchers wanted to see if there would be any sign of vaccine-derived poliovirus (VDPV) afterwards. They included the strains used in the inactivated polio vaccine (IPV) as well, and they took samples from the sewage and analyzed it for polio strains. VDPV strains were found in the sewer systems up to 19 weeks later.[13]

Samples from sewers around the world have been tested and monitored by the WHO[14].

In Belarus some 50 years after the oral polio vaccine was used there, polio strains are still being detected in the sewage systems.

Authors of a paper mentioning the Belarus incidence state:

"[…] genetic exchanges with wild poliovirus and perhaps with nonpoliovirus enteroviruses, are also a natural means of evolution for poliovirus vaccine strains."[15]

Chapter 31: Polio – The controversy continues

[1] Wikipedia. (2018, November 16). Paul Hermann Müller. Retrieved from www.en.wikipedia.org/wiki/Paul_Hermann_M%C3%BCller

[2] The Nobel Prize. (n.d.). *Award ceremony speech*. Retrieved from www.nobelprize.org/prizes/medicine/1948/ceremony-speech/

[3] Amazon. (n.d.). *Jim West*. Retrieved from www.amazon.com/Jim-West/e/B00KDKCBZY/ref=dp_byline_cont_ebooks_1

[4] West, J. (2000). DDT Must Be Bad. *BMJ*, 321: 1403. Retrieved from www.bmj.com/rapid-response/2011/10/30/ddt-must-be-bad

[5] The Alan Mason Chesney Medical Archives of the John Hopkins Medical Institutions. (n.d.). *Henry W. Kumm Collection*. Retrieved from www.medicalarchives.jhmi.edu/papers/kumm.html

[6] www.assets.rockefellerfoundation.org/app/uploads/20150530122203/Annual-Report-1951.pdf p.108

[7] The Center of Disease Control and Prevention. (2017, August 1). *Surveillance Systems to Track Progress Toward Polio Eradication — Worldwide, 2015–2016*. Retrieved from www.cdc.gov/mmwr/volumes/66/wr/mm6613a3.htm#T1_down Table 1.

[8] The Center of Disease Control and Prevention. (2017, August 1). *Surveillance Systems to Track Progress Toward Polio Eradication — Worldwide, 2015–2016*. Retrieved from www.cdc.gov/mmwr/volumes/66/wr/mm6613a3.htm#T1_down Table 2.

[9] The Center of Disease Control and Prevention. (2018, December 10). *About Acute Flaccid Myelitis*. Retrieved from www.cdc.gov/acute-flaccid-myelitis/about-afm.html

[10] Washington State Department of Health. (2018, October). *Acute Flaccid Myelitis (AFM)/Poliomyelitis*. Retrieved from www.doh.wa.gov/Portals/1/Documents/5100/420-068-Guideline-PolioAFM.pdf

[11] Ibid.

[12] The Center of Disease Control and Prevention. (2018, December 10). *AFM Investigation*. Retrieved from www.cdc.gov/acute-flaccid-myelitis/afm-surveillance.html

[13] Esteves-Jaramillo, A., Estívariz, C.F., Peñaranda, S., Richardson, V.L., Reyna, J., Coronel, D.L. ...Pallansch, M.A. (2014). Detection of Vaccine-Derived Polioviruses in Mexico Using Environmental Surveillance. *The Journal of Infectious Diseases*, 210(suppl_1), S315–S323, www.doi.org/10.1093/infdis/jiu183

[14] Haymann, D. (2017, December). *Polio Eradication and Surveillance*. Power Point Presentation presented at the 6th PPG Polio Workshop on Transition Planning and Implementation, Geneva, Switzerland. Retrieved from www.polioeradication.org/wp-content/uploads/2018/01/ppg-ws-presentation-heymann-20171208.pdf and http://polioeradication.org/wp-content/uploads/2018/01/ppg-workshop-report-20171208.pdf

[15] Guillot, S., Caro, V., Cuervo, N., Korotkova, E., Combiescu, M., Persu, A., Aubert-Combiescu, A., Delpeyroux, F., ... Crainic, R. (2000). Natural genetic exchanges between vaccine and wild poliovirus strains in humans. *J Virol*, 74(18), 8434-8443.

CHAPTER 32

India's polio

"Accomplishments don't erase shame, hatred, cruelty, silence, ignorance, discrimination, low self-esteem or immorality. It covers it up, with a creative version of pride and ego."

~Shannon L. Alder *(Author)*

Gates foundation personnel went to Pradesh in India in 2010 or 2011. There were nine or 10 cases of wild polio diagnosed every year out of millions of people, yet the foundation still proceeded with a polio campaign encouraging the use of OPV. Within two years there were 47,500 cases of flaccid paralysis, formerly known as polio. [1]

In a paper published in 2013 the authors start their abstract by stating:

"India's success in eliminating wild polioviruses (WPVs) has been acclaimed globally. Since the last case on January 13, 2011 success has been sustained for two years. By early 2014 India could be certified free of WPV transmission, if no indigenous transmission occurs, the chances of which is considered zero." [2]

While the WHO is working on eliminating both the wild and vaccine-derived polioviruses, we want to know how it's possible to eradicate viruses in India without doing anything about their non-existent sewage systems or polluted water. If sanitary conditions are not improved, do they really think the virus can be eradicated using a live viral vaccine?

We now have a polio vaccine that's known to have the ability to cause vaccine-strain polio and perhaps even AFP.

The story of the poliovirus doesn't end there, however.

235

A person exposed to the vaccine-strain polio has been known to shed the virus for many years or even decades. What shedding the virus in this case means is that an infected person is able to infect others by excreting the poliovirus in their stools. We wonder how many times a virus can evolve and mutate within such a timeframe.

Is the carrier shedding the exact same virus all this time, or is the person shedding mutated variants of the virus? Does it perhaps turn into a more virulent virus which causes paralysis in the individual?

We found a paper that may answer these questions for us.

The author of the paper explains:

> "...These strains can transmit from person to person leading to poliomyelitis outbreaks and can replicate for long periods of time in immunodeficient individuals leading to paralysis or chronic infection, with currently no effective treatment to stop excretion from these patients." [3]

The author continues to describe a patient with poor humoral (acquired) immunity, which is the part of the immunity that produces antibodies. He says this patient "has been excreting type 2 vaccine-derived poliovirus for twenty eight years."[4]

After scientists analyzed the strains he had been excreting, they were able to determine that now, 28 years later, the vaccine strain had become more virulent and dangerous.

We now actually have more "children paralyzed by mutant strains of the polio vaccine" than we have "number of children paralyzed by polio itself."[5]

According to package insert, it's recommended that immunosuppressed people get vaccinated:

> "IPOL vaccine should be used in all patients with immunodeficiency diseases and members of such patients' households when vaccination of such persons is indicated."[6]

It is strange to us that immunodeficient individuals are encouraged to receive a vaccine which has been shown to have the ability to mutate and stay in the body for many years and potentially cause a more dangerous effect than the original disease.

We found an article in the *Indian Journal of Medical Ethics,* where the authors speak their minds about the polio eradication in India.

The abstract states:

> *"[...] while India has been considered polio-free for a year. Perhaps not so surprisingly, there has been a huge increase in non-polio acute flaccid paralysis (NPAFP). In 2011, there were an extra 47,500 new cases of NPAFP. Clinically indistinguishable from polio paralysis but twice as deadly, the incidence of NPAFP was directly proportional to doses of oral polio received. Though this data was collected within the polio surveillance system, it was not investigated.[7]*

So, was India really polio-free? The article provides a breakdown of the US\$8 billion plus spent on vaccinating. The money came from different sources; India alone has spent US\$2.5 billion since 1994. The US spent \$2.5 billion "on world-wide polio eradication" and as you may know, Bill Gates has been a big advocate for eradicating polio. He donated \$1.3 billion on polio eradication in India Rotary international added another \$0.8 billion.[8]

It's worth noting these amounts spent on polio eradication are not in the millions, but rather they are in the billions. What such vast amounts have accomplished, and what they are capable of accomplishing is not lost on the authors of the paper:

> *"From India's perspective the exercise has been extremely costly both in terms of human suffering and in monetary terms. It is tempting to speculate what could have been achieved if the \$2.5 billion spent on attempting to eradicate polio were spent on water and sanitation and routine immunisation."[9]*

We wonder how much is being given to help decontaminate and clean water sources or upgrade sewer systems. Would not the eradication of polio and its many varieties be better controlled if eradication programs included sanitary improvements?

We found a correspondence article in *The Lancet* about serious ethical concerns regarding the new monovalent type 1 oral polio vaccine that WHO helped promote for use in eradicating polio in India.

The article states that:

> "[...] *a new vaccine that was five times more potent than previous vaccines, presumably also with increased likelihood of adverse effects. No informed consent was taken, nor was the public told that the vaccine was experimental. Efforts were made to give the impression that the monovalent vaccine was not new but was just the monovalent vaccine used in the 1960s, before the introduction of the trivalent vaccine."*[10]

Another paper was written about the strain this polio program had on the health care system, highlighting real concerns about the risk of contracting vaccine-associated paralytic polio (VAPP) after receiving the oral polio vaccine.

The paper states:

> "[...] *the number of AFP cases has risen alarmingly all over India. [...] these non-polio AFP cases have a two times higher mortality compared with even WPV cases. [...] it will be difficult to provide a logical explanation to the affected child's parents."*[11]

The authors of that paper show a great concern for the way the eradication program was constructed and the "negative impact on routine healthcare services."

One of the solutions the authors suggest:

> "*Emphasis should be given to improve water and sanitation, thus protecting against the many water-borne diseases and not merely polio."* [12]

We think it's interesting how most of the cases are vaccine-derived, yet the authorities insist the best way to protect ourselves is by getting vaccinated:

> "*In the U.S., the last case of naturally occurring polio was in 1979. Today, despite a worldwide effort to wipe out polio, poliovirus continues to affect children and adults in parts of Asia and Africa."* [13]

The Mayo Clinic continues by clearly stating that "[t]he most effective way to prevent polio is vaccination."[14]

A polio memorandum sent to WHO, UNICEF and the Government of India by a few public health professionals in India, shows how real the concern is.[1516]

According to the Sanofi Pasteur package insert for the IPOL vaccine, the observational studies only lasted for 48 hours after vaccination. As table 2 in the package insert shows us, they observed the infants first six hours after vaccination, then after 24 hours and then at 48 hours.[17]

We can't help but wonder in the event a child dies three days after vaccination whether the death is even considered to be associated with the vaccine. After reading various papers and articles on India's polio eradication program, we feel they are suffering the consequences. The authorities are a little too desperate perhaps?

According to Bill Gates:

> *"Vaccination is pretty special because you can do a vaccination campaign anywhere in the world. All you are doing is gathering women from the villages, getting them the vaccines and asking them to go around and find the children."*[18]

Whatever the intention behind this idea is, we cannot help but see a sinister side where women are being tricked into doing the dirty work by gathering the children and bringing them into the vaccination fold. It's a classic case of vaccinators using the blind to lead the blind. This is not to say their intent is evil or unethical in its origin, but their tactics appear to be shady and manipulative. There is a major lack of transparency regarding vaccinations, and no apparent holistic concern for human beings.

Spending billions of dollars to eradicate one of an infinite number of viruses rather than spending it to clean up the rivers, the sewage and the drinking water doesn't make sense. For many, the water they drink and bathe in comes from the same source. Changing this, surely, will reduce the incidence of exposure to different illnesses and help people build up a stronger immune system.

Chapter 32: India's polio

[1] Vashisht, N. and Puliyel, J. (2012). Polio programme: let us declare victory and move on. *Indian Journal of Medical Ethics*, 9(2), 114-117.

[2] John, T. J., & Vashishtha, V. M. (2013). Eradicating poliomyelitis: India's journey from hyperendemic to polio-free status. *The Indian journal of medical research*, 137(5), 881-94.

[3] G. Dunn. "Twenty-Eight Years of Poliovirus Replication in an Immunodeficient Individual: Impact on the Global Polio Eradication Initiative." *PLOS pathogens* August 27, 2015 www.doi.org/10.1371/journal.ppat.1005114

[4] Dunn, G., Klapsa, D., Wilton, T., Stone, L., Minor, P. D., & Martin, J. (2015). Twenty-Eight Years of Poliovirus Replication in an Immunodeficient Individual: Impact on the Global Polio Eradication Initiative. *PLoS pathogens*, 11(8), e1005114. doi:10.1371/journal.ppat.1005114

[5] National Public Radio, Inc. (NPR). (2017, June 28). *Mutant Strains Of Polio Vaccine Now Cause More Paralysis Than Wild Polio*. Retrieved from www.npr.org/sections/goatsandsoda/2017/06/28/534403083/mutant-strains-of-polio-vaccine-now-cause-more-paralysis-than-wild-polio

[6] The Food and Drug Administration (FDA). (n.d.). *Poliovirus Vaccine Inactivated*. Retrieved from www.fda.gov/downloads/biologicsbloodvaccines/vaccines/approvedproducts/ucm133479.pdf

[7] Vashisht, N. and Puliyel, J. (2012). Polio programme: let us declare victory and move on. *Indian Journal of Medical Ethics*, 9(2), 114-117.

[8] Ibid.

[9] Ibid.

[10] Puliyel, J., Sathyamala, C., and Banerji D. (2007). Protective efficacy of a monovalent oral type 1 poliovirus vaccine. [Correspondence]. *Lancet*, 370(9582), DOI: https://doi.org/10.1016/S0140-6736(07)61075-7

[11] Yadav, K., Rai, S.K., Vidushi, A., and Pandav, C.S. (2009). Intensified pulse polio immunization: Time spent and cost incurred at primary healthcare centre. *The National Medical Journal of India*,) 22(1), 13-17.

[12] Yadav, K., Rai, S.K., Vidushi, A., and Pandav, C.S. (2009). Intensified pulse polio immunization: Time spent and cost incurred at primary healthcare centre. *The National Medical Journal of India*,) 22(1), 13-17.

[13] Mayo Clinic. (2017, December 9). *Polio*. Retrieved from www.mayoclinic.org/diseases-conditions/polio/symptoms-causes/syc-20376512

[14] Ibid.

[15] All India Drug Action Network (AIDAN). (2008, August 12). *Memorandum on Pulse Polio*. Retrieved from www.aidanindia.wordpress.com/2008/08/12/memorandum-on-pulse-polio/

[16] True Democracy Party. (2013, March 28). *PARALYSIS HAUNTS 'POLIO FREE' INDIA: 30 Scientific Studies Showing Link Between Vaccines And Autism.*

Retrieved from www.truedemocracyparty.net/2013/03/paralysis-haunts-polio-free-india-30-scientific-studies-showing-link-between-vaccines-and-autism/
[17] Sanofi Pasteur, (n.d.). Poliovirus Vaccine Inactivated. Retrieved from www.fda.gov/downloads/biologicsbloodvaccines/vaccines/approvedproducts/ucm133479.pdf
[18] CNN. (2011, February 4). *Bill Gates: Vaccine-autism link 'an absolute lie'*. Retrieved from www.cnn.com/2011/HEALTH/02/03/gupta.gates.vaccines.world.health/index.html

CHAPTER 33

Hepatitis B virus—Do babies need the vaccine?

"Before broadcasting for 50-some years, I did TV, played 10 years in the big leagues, won a world championship—and played a big part in that, too, letting the Cardinals inject me with hepatitis. Takes a big man to do that."

~Bob Uecker (American baseball player)

Hepatitis B virus (HBV) enters your body through contact with your bodily fluids and attacks the liver. This way, a pregnant woman can pass it on to her baby during birth. According to the WHO, about 257 million people are hepatitis B surface antigen (HBsAg) positive. WHO also states that 887,000 people died from hepatitis B in 2015.[1]

HBV has a bunch of antigens (proteins) covering its outer surface. A collective name for these proteins is HBsAg. Previously, before it received this name, it was known as the Australian antigen.[2]

This antigen was discovered for the first time in an Australian Aborigine by American researcher Baruch Blumberg, MD, PhD[3]. He won the Nobel Prize for this discovery in 1976[4]. Dr. Blumberg discovered that when a person had become infected with the hepatitis B virus, it could be found in the body both as a part of the whole virus or floating around by itself as a single particle.[5]

Some people were known to be carriers of this 'virus' and were considered to be Au(1) individuals, while those who did not have it were Au(0) individuals.[6] It should therefore not come as a surprise that scientists measure the HBsAg markers on our cells when they are doing research on this particular matter.

There is also something called hepatitis B core antigen (HBcAg). You may recall that when a specific invader, in this case the HBV, enters our body, the very first antibody to be produced is the IgM. In order to know at what stage an infection is, the amount of IgM and IgG antibodies are measured[7]. When our body produces IgM antibodies against the HBV, it's in full attack against the HBcAg.

Let's say you get your blood tested and you appear to have multiple IgM antibodies coded for HBcAg. That means you are actively fighting a hepatitis B infection[8]. If you have been vaccinated with the hepatitis B vaccine, your antibodies will not have the code for HBcAg.

Genetically engineered

The HBV vaccine is genetically engineered. When it's made, some of the HBsAgs are removed from an infected person and attached to a circular (plasmid) DNA of a bacterial or yeast cell. Scientists can add whatever code they want into this plasmid DNA. Usually they add around 15 to 30 genes. They actually have to add whatever is needed in order to keep the new virus alive. [9] For instance, they will add a code for antibiotic resistance. This way, the antibiotic used in the making of the vaccine will not destroy the newly-created DNA.

We now have a new recombined hepatitis B virus, and we need to replicate it. In order to replicate the new virus, it's inserted into a living yeast cell culture for fermentation. The concern about using yeast is that it can cause molecular mimicry. Yeast is very much like the human DNA. Approximately one third of the yeast proteins are the same as ours.

What does that mean when injected into our body?

Here you have substances that are designed to aggravate the immune system towards an attack. And that's what happens. Our immune system launches an attack on the invader, only this invader has many similar protein codes to we humans. Our immune system downloads these protein codes, identifies them as the enemy and starts attacking everything in our body with those specific codes. Unfortunately, our immune system doesn't know how to distinguish between them and our own proteins.

Babies

One concern we see being expressed repeatedly on the Internet is that the hepatitis B vaccine is aimed at fighting a disease infants are rarely exposed to. The chance of infants becoming infected is thought to be miniscule in comparison to their dying or becoming a victim of its many adverse effects.

So, why would we vaccinate newborn babies? According to the World Health Organization (WHO):

> *"Most of the burden of disease from HBV infection comes from infections acquired before the age of 5 years. Therefore, prevention of HBV infection focuses on children under 5 years of age."*[10]

The report continues to explain that in both Africa and Asia, most newborns become infected when their mothers are positive for both HBsAg and HBcAg as opposed to only HBsAg.

They say that:

> *"HBcAg-negative mothers have a near 0% risk of transmitting HBV to their offspring vaccinated at birth, while HBcAg-positive mothers have a 20% risk of transmitting the virus despite vaccination at birth."*[11]

After vaccinating the population in 2015, WHO measured the HBsAg in children under five years of age in the WHO regions. In the African region, they found this antigen in 3% the children and in 1.6% of children in the Eastern Mediterranean region. All other regions were below 1%.[12]

Before the vaccination, WHO claimed 257 million people worldwide had chronic hepatitis B infection. Compared to other regions, Africa and the Western Pacific had the highest prevalence.[13]

Numbers & figures

The CDC released statistics on the various types of hepatitis B in the US child population. The statistics are shown as per population of 100,000 in US in 2015[14]:

Age/Type	Population	Acute	Chronic	Perinatal
<1 yr-olds (per 100K)		1	7	21
1–4 yr-olds (per 100K)		0	17	15
Total in population	19,907,281	199	4,776	7,164
5–14 yr-olds (per 100K)		1	99	0
Total in population	20,171,659	201	19,899	0
(0–14 yr-olds) Total in population	40,078,940	400	24,675	7,164

As at July 2015, there were about 19,907,281 million children under the age of five in the US.[15] Since the data shows the HBV incidences per 100,000 children, we need to multiply by 199 in order to calculated the incidence rate for the entire child population. This means that in the US in 2015, there were 199 children under age five with acute hepatitis B, 4,776 with chronic hepatitis B and 7,164 babies born with hepatitis B. Going with the numbers from the first reference, there were 20,171,659 children in the age group 5–14.[16] In this age group, 201 children had acute hepatitis B, 19,899 had chronic, and 0 had perinatal.

We can see the concern from the medical community's perspective, but how do these statistics compare to the reports submitted to Vaccine Adverse Event Reporting System (VAERS)?

Keep in mind that reporting vaccine reaction to VAERS is extremely rare. Some say as rare as 1% of all cases while others say it's 10% of all cases. Another thing that makes it difficult for us to rely on in VAERS data is that it isn't just medical personnel who can submit data. Parents or others can also submit vaccine reactions children experience. This begs the question whether a child can accidentally be recorded twice.

Another concern is, we found VAERS' search engine not very user-friendly. It was difficult for us who weren't familiar with their website prior to this book, to figure out how to conduct an accurate search. We had difficulty separating adverse reactions per child rather than per symptom. Our most difficult conundrum was when a child is reported having multiple symptoms, how do we know these are all from the same child? Let's say one week it shows 150 reported new events. Are these 150 individual children having their symptoms reported or 50 children all having three reportable events?

With this in mind, we are very reluctant to get into numbers, but we recommend you familiarize yourself with VAERS as it can be useful for those who want to know more about the prevalence of symptoms and to report symptoms. Their website is www.medalerts.org/vaersdb/index.php. If you would like to see the graph and list of symptoms we searched, you can find it here www.medalerts.org/vaersdb/findfield.php.

Chapter 33: Hepatitis B virus – Do babies need the vaccine?
[1] The World Health Organization (WHO). (2018, July 18). *Hepatitis B.* Retrieved from www.who.int/news-room/fact-sheets/detail/hepatitis-b
[2] The Centers for Disease Control and Prevention (CDC). (2017, March 16). *Hepatitis B.* Retrieved from www.cdc.gov/vaccines/pubs/pinkbook/hepb.html
[3] The Nobel Prize. (n.d.). *Baruch S. Blumberg Biographical.* Retrieved from www.nobelprize.org/prizes/medicine/1976/blumberg/auto-biography/
[4] Blumberg, B.S. (1976, December 13). *Australia Antigen and the Biology of Hepatitis B.* Nobel Lecture presented at the Karolinska Institutet, Sweden. Retrieved from www.assets.nobelprize.org/uploads/2018/06/blumberg-lecture.pdf?_ga=2.90778654.542209871.1536107937-250239984.1536107937
[5] History of Vaccines. (n.d.). Retrieved from www.historyofvaccines.org/content/hepatitis-b-australia-antigen
[6] Blumberg, B. S., Friedlaender, J. S., Woodside, A., Sutnick, A. I., & London, W. T. (1969). Hepatitis and Australia antigen: autosomal recessive inheritance of susceptibility to infection in humans. *Proceedings of the National Academy of Sciences of the United States of America*, 62(4), 1108-1115.
[7] Lakna. (2017, October 20). Difference Between Immunoglobulin and Antibody. *Pediaa.* Retrieved from pediaa.com/difference-between-immunoglobulin-and-antibody/
[8] Lymenet. (n.d.). *Current Disease.* Retrieved from www.lymenet.de/labtests/IgMIgGtimes.htm
[9] MacDonald, P.N (Ed.). (2001). *Two-Hybrid Systems: Methods and Protocols.* New Jersey: Humana Press Inc.
[10] The World Health Organization (WHO). (2017). *Global Hepatitis Report, 2017.* Retrieved from www.apps.who.int/iris/bitstream/handle/10665/255016/9789241565455-eng.pdf;jsessionid=4243B9466E2F2681367C7A9561F0A126?sequence=1
[11] Ibid
[12] Ibid.
[13] Ibid.
[14] The Center for Disease Control and Prevention (CDC). (2017, August 11). *Summary of Notifiable Infectious Diseases and Conditions – United States, 2015.* [SeeTable 4]. Retrieved at www.cdc.gov/mmwr/volumes/64/wr/pdfs/mm6453.pdf
[15] United States Census Bureau. (2016, June). *Annual Estimates of the Resident Population by Single Year of Age and Sex for the United States: April 1, 2010 to July 1, 2015. 2015 Population Estimates.* Retrieved from www.factfinder.census.gov/faces/tableservices/jsf/pages/productview.xhtml?pid=PEP_2015_PEPSYASEXN&prodType=table
[16] Ibid.

CHAPTER 34

Hepatitis B virus vaccine—Syndromes

"It does indeed seem absurd that an organic disposition should make beings more fragile, more susceptible to poisons, for in most cases everything in living beings seems disposed to assure them a greater power of resistance."

~Dr. Charles Richet *(French physiologist)*

A new syndrome, one we couldn't find in the VAERS report, is macrophagic myofasciitis (MF or MMF). This syndrome is attributed to the aluminum used in vaccines[1], especially in the hepatitis B vaccine and the tetanus vaccine. Individuals with MF suffer severe pain in their muscles and joints. MRI scans have also shown severe brain injuries.[2]

There have also been cases of multiple sclerosis (MS) after hepatitis B vaccination. In fact, there have been laboratory tests that confirm HBV could cause MS via molecular mimicry. This isn't easy to determine as it can be very difficult to detect the enzymes in question due to their extremely low concentration.[3]

In France, the courts acknowledge multiple sclerosis (MS) can be caused by the vaccine when expressed soon after vaccination, and award compensation to the victims. This has caused quite a stir in the scientific community, which feels the correlation between MS and the HBV vaccine is based "on a hypothetical causal link."[456]

Death by vaccine

The German *Focus magazine* published an article called *Tod in 48 stunden* (Dead in 48 hours). In this study, the researchers found that after random calculation, infants vaccinated with the Hexavac vaccine were 2.5 times more likely to die compared to the average mortality rate.

The researchers also went out of their way to point out that although there is a "temporal connection," they cannot prove there is a causal connection. Therefore, the conclusion was "statistically not significant." This is a common scientific term for not enough proof of relationship between factors. [7]

The above-mentioned study, which was published in 2004, states that 400 infants in Germany die from SIDS.

Although there's awareness of the potential of connection between these events and vaccines, neither the European Medicines Agency nor the Paul Ehrlich Institute recognize a "causal link" between vaccination and death. [8]

On my nerves

We found another very interesting paper on research performed in Guangdong Province, in China, where the researchers looked into the neonatal hepatitis B vaccination.

The researchers conclude:

> "[...] early HBV vaccination induces impairments in behavior and hippocampal neurogenesis. This work provides data supporting the long, suspected potential association of HBV with certain neuropsychiatric disorders such as autism and multiple sclerosis." [9]

Although most hep B vaccines are thimerosal-free now, some countries still have hep B vaccines with thimerosal. A study was done in newborn rhesus macaques (Macaca mulatta) to see how they reacted to thimerosal containing hepatitis B vaccine.

The monkeys were vaccinated within 24 hours of birth and it was found that compared to the monkeys that received either no vaccine or a placebo, the vaccinated monkeys showed "a significant delay" in "three survival reflexes including root, suck and snout [...]."[10]

The researchers also found low birth weight and gestational age intensified the severity of the vaccine reaction. As in some human studies, the researchers observed that the male monkeys reacted more severely than the female monkeys.[11]

This study, as you perhaps can imagine, was highly criticized. Its first publication in 2009 was retracted, but this later publication from 2010 was accepted and to this day has not been retracted. We didn't compare the two versions to see what had changed.

The results from the above macaque study were not very popular and were highly criticized by some vaccine proponents. Authors of a study, which consisted of some of the same authors as the above study, published in 2015 another attempt at similar research.

The main difference between the studies is that in the earlier study from 2010 there were two control groups. One group consisted of four monkeys receiving placebo and the other group of three monkeys receiving no injection at all. The new study from 2015 changed the control group so that 16 monkeys received saline injections.

The results from this study contradicted that of the previous study.

The authors concluded:

> *"This comprehensive 5-year case–control study, which closely examined the effects of pediatric vaccines on early primate development, provided no consistent evidence of neurodevelopmental deficits or aberrant behavior in vaccinated animals."*[12]

Again, these are exactly the type of irregularities that make reviews of vaccine research difficult to compare or assess. Even though the 2015 study above didn't have a large sample size, it did have a larger sample size than the 2010 study.

We also noticed that when the 2010 paper was first published in 2009 (before being revised the following year), Dr. Wakefield, known for the infamous *MMR study[13]*, was listed as one of its authors. When the paper was revised and resubmitted in 2010, his name was no longer listed. We don't know if his name stigmatized the paper and was therefore taken off or if he simply chose not to be a part of the revision. Either way, perhaps a more in-depth look into the research performed in these papers would clarify the discrepancies.

Moving on...

A case study on "children with a first episode of acute CNS inflammatory demyelination in France" from 1994 to 2003 found that:

> *"Hepatitis B vaccination does not generally increase the risk of CNS inflammatory demyelination in childhood. However, the Engerix B vaccine appears to increase this risk, particularly for confirmed multiple sclerosis, in the longer term."[14]*

Data was collected on boys aged 3–17 years of age and born before 1999 who received the neonatal hepatitis B vaccine compared to those who didn't. Those who received the vaccination, according to parental reports, were three times more likely to be diagnosed with autism than those who did not receive the vaccine.[15]

A couple of researchers at Stony Brook University Medical School, at Stony Brook, New York, published a study in 2008 investigating a correlation between the triple series of hepatitis B vaccine and "developmental disability." In their study they included 1,824 children at the ages one to nine years old.

They found that:

> *"The odds of receiving EIS [special education services] were approximately nine times as great for vaccinated boys (n = 46) as for unvaccinated boys (n = 7), [...]."[16]*

Trial by no jury

We find it very concerning that the clinical safety trials for our vaccines are based on only a few days of observations.

It is widely stated in multiple research studies that it can take several months for symptoms to appear after being vaccinated. For instance, with the Recombivax HB vaccine there were three clinical studies performed on 147 healthy infants lasting only five days. We also know now that when researchers specify *healthy* infants, we can expect that children with a weaker immune system would have been excluded. This would not be a true assessment of those who receive the vaccine as a part of the vaccine schedule.

Another concern with their study of 147 *healthy* children is as mentioned earlier, if we are to assume that serious events are extremely rare, say as low as one in 10,000, then how can such events possibly be determined by studying 147 infants and children over a five-day period?[17]

Not only did they select healthy infants and children, but they failed to include a control group. Based on these studies, do the CDC and the FDA really know how safe these vaccines are?

Too much metal

According to John Hopkins website for vaccine safety, information written in 2000 states that "[t]he new Engerix-B contains only trace amounts of thimerosal (≤1 mcg)"[18].

This is interesting considering what we found in a paper written five years later, in 2005, which states:

> *"Studies in preterm infants indicate that blood levels of Hg after just one vaccination (hepatitis B) increase by >10-fold to levels above the US EPA guidelines."*[19]

253

It's not just the mercury or the genetic engineering of DNA from different species that has many people concerned about the HepB vaccine. The concern that side effects could be coming from the immense amount of aluminum being dispensed has also been expressed.

A hepatitis B vaccine dose for newborns has 250 mcg of aluminum. The limit should not exceed five mcg/kg. If a baby weighs five kilos, that's 5kg x 5mcg = 25 mcg. This means we are injecting ten times the possibly safe dose of known toxin into children. To us this appears to be a guaranteed way for a tiny body to accumulate aluminum.

And this is just the start. It's sobering when you stop to think these vaccines containing aluminum will continue to be administered for years to come.

Chapter 34: Hepatitis B virus vaccine – Syndromes

[1] Bonnefont-Rousselot, D., Chantalat-Auger, C., Teixeira, A., Jaudon, M.C, Pelletier, S., and Cherin, P. (2004). Blood oxidative status in patients with macrophagic myofasciitis. *Biomed Pharmacol*, 58(9), 516-519.

[2] Authier, F.J., Cherin, P., Creange, A., Bonnotte, B., Ferrer, X., Abdelmoumni, A., ...Gherardi, R.K. (2001). Central nervous system disease in patients with macrophagic myofasciitis. *Brain*, 124(Pt 5), 974-983

[3] Faure, E. (2005). Multiple sclerosis and hepatitis B vaccination: could minute contamination of the vaccine by partial hepatitis B virus polymerase play a role through molecular mimicry? *Med Hypotheses*, 65(3), 509-520.

[4] Rougé-Maillart, C.l., Guillaume, N., Jousset, N., and Penneau, M. (2007). Recognition by French courts of compensation for post-vaccination multiple sclerosis: the consequences with regard to expert practice. *Med Sci Law*, 47(3), 185-190.

[5] Vogel, G. (2017, June 27). Decision by Europe's top court alarms vaccine experts. *Science*. Retrieved from www.sciencemag.org/news/2017/06/decision-europe-s-top-court-alarms-vaccine-experts

[6] Schipani, V. (2017, July 3). Scientific Evidence and the EU Court. *FactCheck.org*. Retrieved from www.factcheck.org/2017/07/scientific-evidence-eu-court/

[7] Schauttauer, G. (2004, October 18). Tod in 48 Stunden. *Focus Magazin* Nr. 43. Retrieved from www.focus.de/politik/deutschland/studie-tod-in-48-stunden_aid_201268.html

[8] Ibid.

[9] Yang, J., Qi, F., Yang, Y., Yuan, Q., Zou, J., Guo, K., and Yao, Z. (2016). Neonatal hepatitis B vaccination impaired the behavior and neurogenesis of mice transiently in early adulthood. *Psychoneuroendocrinology*, 73, 166-176.

[10] Hewitson, L., Houser, L.A, Carol, S., Sackett, G., Tomko, J.L, Atwood, D., ...White, E.R. (2010). Delayed acquisition of neonatal reflexes in newborn primates receiving a thimerosal-containing Hepatitis B vaccine: Influence of gestational age and birth weight. *Journal of Toxicology and Environmental Health, Part A*, 73(19), 1298-1313

[11] Ibid.

[12] Curtis, B., Liberato, N., Rulien, M., Morrisroe, K., Kenney, C., Yutuc, V., Ferrier, C., Marti, C. N., Mandell, D., Burbacher, T. M., Sackett, G. P., ... Hewitson, L. (2015). Examination of the safety of pediatric vaccine schedules in a non-human primate model: assessments of neurodevelopment, learning, and social behavior. Environmental health perspectives, 123(6), 579-589.

[13] Wakefield, A.J., Murch, S.H., Anthony, A., Linnell, J., Casson, D.M., Malik, M., ... Walker-Smith, J.A. (1998). Ileal-lymphoid-nodular hyperplasia, non-specific colitis, and pervasive developmental disorder in children. *The Lancet*, 351(9103), P637-641.

[14] Mikaeloff, Y., Caridade, G., Suissa, S., and Tardieu, M. (2009). Hepatitis B vaccine and the risk of CNS inflammatory demyelination in childhood. *Neurology*, 72(10), 873-880. doi: 10.1212/01.wnl.0000335762.42177.07.

[15] Gallagher, C.M. and Goodman, M.S. (2010). Hepatitis B vaccination of male neonates and autism diagnosis, NHIS 1997-2002. *J Toxicol Environ Health A*, 73(24), 1665-1677.

[16] Gallagher, C. and Goodman, M. (2008). Hepatitis B triple series vaccine and developmental disability in US children aged 1-9 years. *Toxicological & Environmental Chemistry*, 90(5), 997–1008.

[17] The Food and Drug Administration (FDA). (n.d.). *Recombivax Hepatitis B vaccine.* Retrieved from www.fda.gov/downloads/BiologicsBloodVaccines/Vaccines/ApprovedProducts/UCM110114.pdf

[18] John Hopkins Bloomberg School of Public Health (2017, October 18). Preservative-Free Hepatitis B Vaccine. Retrieved from www.vaccinesafety.edu/news-SKB%20no-preserv-hepb-vax.htm

[19] Burbacher, T. M., Shen, D. D., Liberato, N., Grant, K. S., Cernichiari, E., & Clarkson, T. (2005). Comparison of blood and brain mercury levels in infant monkeys exposed to methylmercury or vaccines containing thimerosal. *Environmental health perspectives*, 113(8), 1015-1021.

CHAPTER 35

Hepatitis A virus vaccine—How badly do we need it?

"Water, air, and cleanness are the chief articles in my pharmacy."

~Napoléon Bonaparte (French statesman and military leader)

Another hepatitis virus children are vaccinated for is the hepatitis A virus. Humans are the only ones to fall sick after contracting this virus. Other primates can contract it and transfer it over to humans, but it doesn't actually infect other primates. The virus is excreted with the feces and that's how it transfers from one human to another. For instance, imagine if someone who's infected and is working at a fast food restaurant doesn't wash his or her hands. As you eat the burger and fries they made and drink the Coke they poured complete with the ice they scooped with bare hands, the virus travels into your intestines.

As comedian Adam Carolla said, "Mmm, tastes like hepatitis!"[1]

As you know, your gut, is permeable. The virus is able to penetrate the gut-brain barrier and enter the bloodstream. From there it reaches the liver and then attacks the liver cells, the virus replicates and sends its "offspring" into the bile. The bile is now covered in viruses, which are flushed out with the feces.

The hepatitis A virus can survive on surfaces outside the body for several days. According to a Canadian study published in 2000, hepatitis A:

> *"[...] can readily survive freezing, persist in fresh or salt water for up to 12 months and can retain its infectivity for a few days to weeks in dried feces."*[2]

Once you have become infected with the virus, there is no treatment for it. Usually a treatment wouldn't be necessary anyway since 99% of those who become infected with the virus recover on their own.

The CDC says that:

> *"Symptoms of hepatitis A can include:*
>
> *"fever, fatigue, loss of appetite, nausea, vomiting, and/or joint pain*
>
> *"severe stomach pains and diarrhea (mainly in children), or*
>
> *"jaundice [...]*
>
> *"Children often do not have symptoms, but most adults do. [...]*
>
> *"Hepatitis A can cause liver failure and death, although this is rare and occurs more commonly in persons 50 years of age or older and persons with other liver diseases [...]."*[3]

What does the WHO say?

> *"Almost everyone recovers fully from hepatitis A with a lifelong immunity. However, a very small proportion of people infected with hepatitis A could die from fulminant hepatitis.*
>
> *"Those infected in childhood do not experience any noticeable symptoms. Epidemics are uncommon because older children and adults are generally immune."*[4]

Okay, maybe we're just a couple of novices, but let's look at this for a second. When children become infected with hepatitis A they are extremely unlikely to have any noticeable symptoms. In fact, according to the WHO, no children experience noticeable symptoms. It also states that these children who become infected carry a lifelong immunity. If you become infected when you're older, you are more likely to become seriously ill to the point of liver failure or death.

Then why are we vaccinating children with a vaccine that doesn't provide lifelong immunity, especially considering the disease itself is quite safe and clears up on its own? When they grow older and the vaccine wanes, they are in danger of becoming seriously ill from a disease they wouldn't even know they had, if given the chance to become naturally infected at a young age.

The making of

The HepA vaccine is an inactivated whole virus vaccine. It's grown in MRC-5 human cell culture. After the germ has grown in the culture media, the virus is attenuated using formaldehyde. It is now incapable of replicating any further. Although the virus is inactive, it's still a whole virus. This is important in order for our immune system to recognize it as such and react to the invasion.

In short: in order to grow and inactivate the hepatitis A virus for vaccine use, human cell cultures and formaldehyde are used for the process.

Side effects

The problem with finding this vaccine's specific side effects is that it is rarely, if ever, dispensed on its own. We feel that, as with most other vaccines, it is more the fact that it adds to the accumulative effect from multiple vaccines. This factor may also make it very difficult to pinpoint a vaccine as the cause of adverse effects in court cases. Perhaps that's why not many cases even make it to court.

Researching how the adverse events from the vaccine looked compared to the effects of the natural illness, we ended up on a page created by the National Vaccine Injury Compensation Program (NVIC) where they listed the cases filed in court from 1988–2017. Although it says it covers the period from 1988, the Hepatitis A vaccines were not included in the compensation program until December 1, 2004.[5] Cases filed relate to 97 injuries and seven deaths attributed specifically to the Hep A vaccines. It doesn't specify which cases were dismissed, compensated or settled.[6]

Although the vaccine is rumored to be linked with autism, there's *no direct evidence* that it, or any other vaccine, causes autism. *However,* it has been pointed out that autism rates are linked with the use of human fetal cells in the vaccines. Hepatitis A contains human fetal cells and so do other vaccines given at the same time. So, there would be a higher concentration of human DNA contaminants being injected during the same doctor visit.

Chapter 35: Hepatitis A virus vaccine – how badly do we need it?
[1] Carolla, A. and Kimmel, J. (1999-2014) The Man Show. Retrieved from
www.imdb.com/title/tt0202741/characters/nm0453994
[2] Sattar, S. A., Jason, T., Bidawid, S., & Farber, J. (2000). Foodborne spread of
hepatitis A: Recent studies on virus survival, transfer and inactivation. *The
Canadian journal of infectious diseases = Journal canadien des maladies infectieuses*, 11(3),
159-163.
[3] Centers for Disease Control and Prevention (CDC). (2016, July 20). *Hepatitis A
VIS*. Retrieved from www.cdc.gov/vaccines/hcp/vis/vis-statements/hep-a.html
[4] World Health Organization (WHO). (2018, September 19). *Hepatitis A*. Retrieved
from www.who.int/news-room/fact-sheets/detail/hepatitis-a
[5] Department of Health and Human Services. (2004, December 1). *National
Vaccine Injury Compensation Program: Inclusion of Hepatitis A Vaccines in the Vaccine in the
injury Table*. [Vol. 69, No. 230]. Retrieved from www.gpo.gov/fdsys/pkg/FR-2004-
12-01/pdf/04-26273.pdf
[6] National Vaccine Injury Compensation Program. (2017, November 28). *Data &
Statistics*. [Monthly Statistics Report].
www.nvic.org/cmstemplates/nvic/pdf/vicp/vicp-monthly-report-12-2017.pdf

CHAPTER 36

H. influenzae type b vaccine—No, it's not the flu

"Is it not meningitis?"

*~Author Louisa May Alcott's last words after
she had fallen ill and become invalid.*

During the influenza outbreak in 1892, which occurred before the discovery of influenza virus, a group of sick individuals were diagnosed with the flu. It was later realized these patients didn't have the flu at all, but something else entirely: a bacterial infection. But, because of the timing and association with the influenza outbreak, scientists called the germ *Haemophilus influenzae* type b (Hib).

Hib causes numerous complications and is the most common cause of bacterial meningitis. It also causes neurological damages and pneumonia. Once a person is infected with Hib it can become a very serious illness. What makes the Hib strain so virulent is its slimy, protective polysaccharide capsule called PRP.

A surveillance study done in Salvador, Brazil, examined how effective the Hib vaccine was. The vaccine was put into use in August 1999, and a year later, Hib meningitis cases had gone from 2.62 cases per 100,000 individuals to 0.81 cases per 100,000 individuals.[1]

There was only one problem. *H. influenzae* type a (Hia) meningitis had the opportunity to grow where it otherwise wouldn't have, and it went from 0.02 cases per 100,000 individuals to 0.16 cases per 100,000 individuals. This may not seem like many cases, but if you look at the increase (in cases), they were now eight times higher.

The increase in non-hib cases sparked interest in other researchers. Authors of a 2011 paper analyzed samples that had been sent to the National Reference Laboratory (NRL)[2] in the period between 1990 and

2008. Before the vaccine was introduced in August 1999, Hib accounted for 98% of all *H. influenzae* meningitis cases. After the vaccine was introduced, it had dropped to 59%, meaning, yes, the vaccine was working, but instead other *H. influenzae* strains had begun to take its place.

The Brazilian Ministry of Health considered the data from its national laboratory to show "that Hib meningitis has been effectively controlled in Brazil using a 3-dose schedule in the first year of life without a booster."[3]

Because the Hib vaccine uses the bacterial sugar coat (PRP) rather than the actual germ, it is unable to cause disease. So, just like the Hepatitis B vaccine, it needs to be attached to a carrier protein in order to aggravate the immune system. Each vaccine manufacturer differs in the way they have decided to go about this process.

Another surveillance study, covering the period 1983 through 2011 and this time performed in Alaska, focused on the indigenous population of this US state. The researchers focused on this group because the indigenous people appeared to have the highest Hib disease rate in the world.

The vaccine was first introduced to Alaska's native population in 1991. Unfortunately, the same thing happened there as occurred in China. While the vaccine successfully reduced the number of Hib cases, *Haemophilus influenzae* type a (Hia) rose. Prior to 2002, the Alaskan indigenous population had not had a single diagnosed case of Hia, but between 2002 and 2011 there were 32 diagnoses of Hia.

The authors of that study state:

> *"Since the introduction of the Hib conjugate vaccine, Hia infection has become a major invasive bacterial disease in Alaska Native children."*[4]

A deviation from Hib strain has also been observed in Ontario, Canada. They are seeing *Haemophilus influenzae* type f (Hif) and non-typable strains. A non-typable strain is a strain that has not been identified as a specific type, such as type a or b or f. In adults, this seems to have become a more serious disease and often presents itself in the form of sepsis.[5] Sepsis is when bacteria infect your blood. In order to defend itself your body starts an inflammatory process, which may lead to the shutdown of organs.

Similar results were observed in Utah. After an epidemiological study spanning a decade, from 1998–2008, it was noticed that while the Hib disease decreased in children, the adult population was experiencing an increase in and a more serious *H. influenzae* disease. As with the Canada study, "*H. influenzae* disease was attributable to an increase in nontypable and Hif strains."[6]

The body reacts

Allergic reactions have been seen as a result of the Hib vaccine. In the book *the Peanut Allergy Epidemic* the author mentions how the Hib bacterium has proteins so similar to the peanut molecular structure that it causes our body to make antibodies against peanuts. This has the potential to become peanut allergy in the vaccinated individual.[7]

Another disease that has been tied to the Hib vaccine is Insulin Dependent Diabetes Mellitus (IDDM). A study published in 2002 was done in Finland to see if this association was valid. Researchers used the data from a clinical trial, which included 116,000 children born between October 1st and August 31st, who each received four doses of the Hib vaccine. The control group consisted of 128,500 children who were born two years before the vaccine was released, and therefore did not receive it. The researchers conclude that "[e]xposure to HiB immunization is associated with an increased risk of IDDM."[8]

These results were supported in a Swedish study where it was found the HiB vaccine increased the risk of diabetes by affecting the "beta cell-related immune response" through stimulating the GADA and 1A-2A production.[9] (GADA are autoantibodies that attack a certain enzyme in the beta cells that produce insulin. 1A-2A are also autoantibodies that attack a specific enzyme in the beta cells).

According to the National Centre for Immunisation Research & Surveillance (NCIRS), the association between HiB and diabetes is flawed.

In fact, they state:

> *"The highly respected international Cochrane Collaboration reviewed all the available studies and did not find an increased risk of diabetes associated with vaccination."* [10]

They were not the only ones to come to this conclusion:

> *"Expert groups such as the National Institutes of Health in the USA have met and reviewed the evidence and conclude that there is no link between vaccines and diabetes."*[11]

Mind you, the Cochrane Collaboration, which we generally highly respect, did not find any correlation between aluminum and the DTP vaccine either and they shut down their entire vaccine research program. Despite this, we acknowledge that NCIRS is a highly respected organization in the scientific community, known for its research reviews and believed to be independent of financial or other pecuniary interests.

As with other vaccines, the safety studies performed for the Hib vaccine only observed their subjects for three or four days. So, upon reviewing these studies it would be difficult to come to any other conclusions when contradictory or conflicting data is simply unavailable.

When it comes to autoimmune or neurological diseases, three to four days is often not long enough to determine whether a correlation between a substance and a vaccine is occurring.

We feel there's grounds for suspicion that many of the children with allergies today may have them as a result of receiving vaccinations.

Chapter 36: H. influenzae type b vaccine – No, it's not the flu

[1] Riberio, G.S., Reis, J.N., Cordeiro, S,M., Lima, J.B., Gouveia, E.L., Petersen, M., …Ko, A.l. (2003). Prevention of *Haemophilus influenzae* type b (Hib) Meningitis and Emergence of Serotype Replacement with Type a Strains after Introduction of Hib Immunization in Brazil. *The Journal of Infectious Diseases*, 187(1), 109-116 ·

[2] National Reference Laboratory. (n.d.). *About Us*. Retrieved from https://nrl.ae/en/contents/view/about-us.html

[3] Zanella, R.C., Bokermann, S., Andrade, A.L., Flannery, B., and Brandileone, M.C. (2011). Changes in serotype distribution of Haemophilus influenzae meningitis isolates identified through laboratory-based surveillance following routine childhood vaccination against H. influenzae type b in Brazil. *Vaccine*, 29(48), 8937-8942.

[4] Bruce, M.G., Zulz, T., DeByle, C., Singleton, R., Hurlburt, D., Bruden, D., …Wenger, J.D. (2013). Haemophilus influenzae Serotype a Invasive Disease, Alaska, USA, 1983–2011. *Emerging Infectious Diseases*, 19(6), 932-937.

[5] Adams, H.J., Richardson, S.E., Jamieson, F.B., Rawte, P., Low, D.E., and Fisman, D.N. (2010). Changing epidemiology of invasive Haemophilus influenzae in Ontario, Canada: evidence for herd effects and strain replacement due to Hib vaccination. *Vaccine*, 28(24), 4073-4078.

[6] Rubach, M. P., Bender, J. M., Mottice, S., Hanson, K., Weng, H. Y., Korgenski, K., Daly, J. A., … Pavia, A. T. (2011). Increasing incidence of invasive Haemophilus influenzae disease in adults, Utah, USA. *Emerging infectious diseases*, 17(9), 1645-1650.

[7] Frasier, H.A. (2011). *The peanut allergy epidemic: what's causing it and how to stop it*. [p. 7.]. New York, NY: Skyhorse Pub.

[8] Classen, J.B. and Classen, D.C. (2002). Clustering of cases of insulin dependent diabetes (IDDM) occurring three years after hemophilus influenza B (HiB) immunization support causal relationship between immunization and IDDM. *Autoimmunity*, 35(4), 247-253

[9] Wahlberg, J., Fredriksson, J., Vaarala, O., Ludvigsson, J., and Abis Study Group. (2003). Vaccinations may induce diabetes-related autoantibodies in one-year-old children. *Ann N Y Acad Sci*, 1005, 404-408.

[10] National Centre for Immunisation Research & Surveillance. (2009, December). *Diabetes and vaccines*. [Fact Sheet]. Retrieved from www.ncirs.org.au/sites/default/files/2018-12/diabetes-and-vaccines-fact-sheet.pdf

[11] Ibid.

CHAPTER 37

Meningococcal vaccine—The many shades

"No infectious disease is more terrifying to parents than that caused by meningococcus."

~Paul Offit (Vaccines. What you should know. p.131)

Meningococcal disease is caused by a germ called *Neisseria meningitidis*. It can cause, among other things, bacterial meningitis, which is an infection of the membrane covering the brain and the spinal cord. This is very rare, but if you become infected, there is a chance you'll suffer complications such as mental retardation.

In 2015 there was a meningitis outbreak at the University of Oregon, in Eugene, Oregon, US. There were seven students who were confirmed infected. One died. Because the germ is spread through sneezing and coughing, it's easy for the germ to find new hosts—especially when people are in close vicinity in dorm rooms and the like.

If you catch it early enough, the germ can be treated with antibiotics before it causes any damage. Being able to recognize abnormal behavior or symptoms in your child can be vital as early medical intervention is required before the germ reaches the nerves or the brain.

As with so many other germs, this one has multiple strains. There are 12 serogroups that we know of, and half of them (A, B, C, W, X, Y) have been known to cause epidemics[1]. Almost one third of all cases are caused by serogroup B. Unfortunately, the childhood vaccines do not protect against serogroup B.

In most industrialized countries, Meningococcal meningitis is very rare. In 2016 in the US, 90 cases were recorded in children age 0–15 years.[2]

According to The World Bank data, the child population in the age group 0–14 was approximately 61,000,000.[3] This is not taking into account all the 15-year-olds as they are combined with a different population group. Ignoring this error, as we are unable to add them to our calculations, about one child in every 677,000 is infected with Meningococcal meningitis. Out of the 90 infected, 11 children died. So, as you can see, although this disease is not very common, it is quite serious and has a high death rate.

The most common vaccines used in the US are Menactra and Menveo. They cover the serogroups A, C, W and Y.[4] When it comes to the age group 0–15, out of the 90 cases, 50 of them were caused by serogroup B and 6 in the non-groupable serotypes.

So, let's look at this again.... out of the 90 cases of meningococcus illnesses in 2016, the vaccine potentially covered, at the most, 34 of those cases. Using the same calculations as in above paragraph, we are now down to about one sick child in every 1.8 million children. This is the worst-case scenario, as, unfortunately, the death rate table does not specify the serogroups contributing to the number of deaths.

Those in many Third World countries are not so lucky. Some African countries are perhaps worst affected. According to the WHO website:

> *"Every year, bacterial meningitis epidemics affect more than 400 million people living in the 26 countries of the extended 'African meningitis belt' [...]."*[5]

In the period 1995–2014, there were 900,000 reported cases of meningococcus illnesses in Africa where 90,000 people died and 90,000–180,000 people suffered neurological damage.[6]

It goes without saying this is quite a serious illness in Africa. However, we are unsure whether the medical authorities tested, or are performing serological testing on those infected in the African population the same way they are in the industrialized countries.

Do they know what is causing the bacterial meningitis in Africa? We ask this because there are different serotypes, which means we don't know how effective the vaccine would be for the African population; and there are other germs that cause meningitis as well.

There are many types of meningitis caused by different organisms such as Hib and streptococcus species, including group B streptococcus. The strain we are concerned about in adolescents and young adults is caused by the bacteria *Neisseria meningitidis,* specifically in the serogroup B. These deadly bacteria can kill within hours.

Other epidemics throughout the world are documented on the WHO's website.[7] Most occur in Africa, but in 2005 epidemics were registered in India[8] and the Philippines.[9] Other epidemics outside of the African continent occurred in 2000. The countries involved then were "Singapore, Indonesia, Iran and Morocco[10], US[11], France, United Kingdom, Oman, Saudi Arabia and Netherlands.[12]

Side effects

In searching for multiple vaccine trials, we turned to the book *Adverse Effects of Vaccines: Evidence and Causality.*[13] In the section on the meningococcal vaccine, multiple side effects were considered and accompanying trial studies analyzed. These adverse effects were, as listed in Table 11–1: encephalitis, encephalopathy, acute disseminated encephalomyelitis (ADEM), transverse myelitis (TM), multiple sclerosis (MS), Guillain-Barré syndrome (GBS), chronic inflammatory disseminated polyneuropathy (CIDP), anaphylaxis and chronic headache.[14]

For every single trial study analysis, the conclusion was either insufficient, limited, lacking or inadequate.[15] There was only one study that provided sufficient data to support a hypothesis or conclusion, and this was in the analysis of trials looking into the correlation between the vaccine and anaphylaxis. The authors of the book state:

> *"The evidence convincingly supports a causal relationship between meningococcal vaccine and anaphylaxis."*[16]

Scientists conduct vaccine trials on vaccines which are designed to be injected into every single child world over. How is it that the best studies medical authorities can come up with consists of insufficient data, which at best is biased, insomuch that their results are unreliable?

In what other scientific fields would this be acceptable?

Chapter 37: Meningococcal vaccine – The many shades
[1] World Health Organization. (2018, February 19). *Meningococcal meningitis.* [Fact sheet]. Retrieved from www.who.int/news-room/fact-sheets/detail/meningococcal-meningitis
[2] Centers for Disease Control and Prevention (CDC). (2017, September). *Enhanced Meningococcal Disease Surveillance Report, 2016.* [Surveillance Report]. Retrieved from www.cdc.gov/meningococcal/downloads/NCIRD-EMS-Report.pdf
[3] The World Bank. (2017). *Population ages 0-14 (% of total).* Retrieved from www.data.worldbank.org/indicator/SP.POP.0014.TO.ZS
[4] Immunization Action Coalition (IAC). (n.d.). *Meningococcal ACWY.* Retrieved from www.immunize.org/askexperts/experts_meningococcal_acwy.asp
[5] World Health Organization (WHO). (n.d.). *Global Health Observatory (GHO) data.* Retrieved from www.who.int/gho/epidemic_diseases/meningitis/en/
[6] Ibid.
[7] World Health Organization (WHO). (n.d.). *Emergency preparedness, response.* Retrieved from www.who.int/csr/don/archive/disease/meningococcal_disease/en/
[8] World Health Organization (WHO). (2005, June 14). *Global Alert and Response (GAR).* Retrieved from www.who.int/csr/don/2005_06_14/en/
[9] World Health Organization (WHO). (2005, January 28). *Emergency preparedness, response.* Retrieved from www.who.int/csr/don/2005_01_28a/en/
[10] World Health Organization (WHO). (2000, May 03). *Emergency preparedness, response.* Retrieved from www.who.int/csr/don/2000_05_03/en/
[11] World Health Organization (WHO). (2000, April 26). *Emergency preparedness, response.* Retrieved from www.who.int/csr/don/2000_04_26/en/
[12] World Health Organization (WHO). (2000, April 21). *Emergency preparedness, response.* Retrieved from www.who.int/csr/don/2000_04_21b/en/
[13] Stratton, K., Ford, A., Rusch, E., and Clayton, E.W. (2011). Meningococcal Vaccine. In Committee to Review Adverse Effects of Vaccines; Institute of Medicine (Eds.). *Adverse Effects of Vaccines: Evidence and Causality.* Washington (DC): National Academies Press (US). ISBN-13: 978-0-309-21435-3ISBN-10: 0-309-21435-1 Retrieved from www.nap.edu/read/13164/chapter/1
[14] Stratton, K., Ford, A., Rusch, E., and Clayton, E.W. (2011). *Adverse Effects of Vaccines: Evidence and Causality.* Committee to Review Adverse Effects of Vaccines; Institute of Medicine (Eds.). (p. 611). Washington (DC): National Academies Press (US). ISBN-13: 978-0-309-21435-3ISBN-10: 0-309-21435-1 Retrieved from www.nap.edu/read/13164/chapter/13#611
[15] Ibid.
[16] Stratton, K., Ford, A., Rusch, E., and Clayton, E.W. (2011). *Adverse Effects of Vaccines: Evidence and Causality.* Committee to Review Adverse Effects of Vaccines; Institute of Medicine (Eds.). (p. 610). Washington (DC): National Academies Press (US). ISBN-13: 978-0-309-21435-3ISBN-10: 0-309-21435-1 Retrieved from www.nap.edu/read/13164/chapter/13#609

CHAPTER 38

Pneumococcal vaccine—The many shades of Prevnar

*"I have a public bathroom rating system that
I keep in my head, and anything that I think
rates lower than two stars, I won't even enter."*

~ **Sally J. Pla** *(The Someday Birds)*

Streptococcus pneumoniae are a family of organisms that many people have been infected by at some point in their lives. This family (strep) has at least 90 different strains of the bacterium called pneumococcus.

Every year, pneumococcus is responsible for a wide range of medical problems in the US, including bacterial pneumonia, bacteremia, ear infections in infants and young children and, as discussed in previous chapter, bacterial meningitis.

Although ear infections are extremely common in young children, the FDA announced that the new vaccine prevents blood poisoning and meningitis, but not ear infections. A person becomes infected when they inhale the droplets that are shed into the air by an already infected individual. Once a person has become infected, the bacteria then enters the bloodstream. From there it can travel to the brain or lungs. Those who have weak immune system may suffer secondary complications like pneumonia.

The pneumococci bacteria live as normal biota in the throat and nose of some individuals. These individuals don't become sick (from the bacteria) nor do they need treatment because the bacteria don't cause disease. Those individuals who don't have it as normal biota in their throat and nose, and instead become sick, are treated with antibiotics. Normally, it only takes about two days or less to get better.

There are two types of pneumococcal vaccines used in the US today.

These are the pneumococcal conjugate vaccine (PCV or Prevnar) and the pneumococcal polysaccharide vaccine (PPSV or Pneumovax).

According to the CDC website, the PPSV should not be given to "children younger than 2 years old" and for those children older than two, this vaccine should only be administered if the child has "certain medical conditions."[1]

As for the PCV vaccine, the CDC recommends that "all children younger than 2 years old" should receive it. For children older than two, the vaccine should only be given for those "with certain medical conditions."[2]

We found this very interesting because when we looked at the website for Mount Sinai Hospital in Toronto, Canada, according to their microbiology department, the vaccine is "for those at high risk of serious infection."[3] Although their website doesn't mention a vaccine by name, the site is "made possible through an unrestricted educational grant from Pfizer Canada Inc."[4] Pfizer is the manufacturer of the Prevnar vaccines.

The webpage continues:

> *"The vaccine is not recommended for children < 2 years as they do not respond satisfactorily. It is not recommended for prevention of inner ear infections of childhood."*[5]

The Mount Sinai Hospital website also points out the specific conditions or illnesses a child must have in order to receive the vaccine. This seems contradictory. It appears the page may not have been updated recently. In the hope of clarifying this, we visited *Pfizer Canada's* website. On their webpage, they state that as of December 2009, 120 countries have approved the use of Prevnar 13 in infants and children.[6]

Their American website confirms the use of the vaccine for infants as young as six weeks old. Here, they also state that since 2016, the vaccine Prevnar 13 includes some of the strains that cause ear infection in infants and children.[7] Their Canadian webpage states, as mentioned above, that as of December 2009 the vaccine was approved for infants and children in 120 countries. The American website, states that as of 2016 the vaccine has been used for infants and children in over 150 countries.

Pfizer prides itself in "[m]anufacturing and delivering world-class vaccines"[8] and explains that:

> *"[...] one dose of Prevenar 13 requires 580 manufacturing*

> *steps, over 1,700 employees, 678 quality tests, 400
> different raw materials, and more than two-and-a-half
> years to manufacture from start to finish."*[9]

The vaccine is called Prevnar and the number accompanying the name shows how many serotypes/strains are included in the vaccine.

You can probably already guess what one of the concerns are when a vaccine only covers a fraction of the strains of a certain bacterium. One research paper that brings up such a concern is a paper written in 2007 with the purpose:

> *"[t]o monitor continuing shifts in the strains of
> Streptococcus pneumoniae that cause AOM [acute otitis
> media] [...] following the introduction of a pneumococcal
> 7-valent conjugate vaccine (PCV7)."*[10]

The authors found that:

> *"In the years following introduction of PCV7, a strain of
> S. pneumoniae has emerged in the United States as an
> otopathogen that is resistant to all FDA-approved
> antibiotics for treatment of AOM in children."*[11]

The vaccine approved for children is the Prevnar vaccine. This is, as mentioned above, a conjugate vaccine. Its bacterial sugar coat is grown in soy peptone (protein derivative) broth. A carrier protein is grown in a strain from the *C. diphtheriae* bacteria in a culture made with bovine protein fragments and yeast products. Because the bacterial sugar coat is too weak to awaken the immune cells, it's attached to a carrier protein. The carrier protein is much stronger and can aggravate the immune cells. Vaccines that are conjugate vaccines are the vaccines for Hepatitis B, Hib, HPV, pneumococcus and meningococcus.

Ever-changing vaccine

As mentioned above, the pneumococcal family has multiple strains. It was unrealistic for the scientists to make a vaccine that covers all the strains. Instead they picked seven strains and introduced Prevnar 7 to the public. It was a vaccine intended to combat seven out of more than 90 different pneumococcal strains.

Within a few years of targeting these seven strains, the vaccine successfully prevented people from getting sick. As with most things, nature finds its way around obstacles or finds a way to take advantage of them. With these seven strains out of harm's way, people started getting sick from different strains. These new strains, which had not caused problems in the past, became more prevalent and more dangerous than those they replaced.

In order to keep up, scientists added six additional strains to the Prevnar vaccine. It became Prevnar 13 instead of Prevnar 7. Within a couple of years, these little microorganisms quickly adapted. There are now already new strains taking the place of these 13 strains.

It appears that each time a pneumococcal vaccine is marketed, other serotypes (strains) keep becoming disease-causing. This makes the vaccine less effective against these diseases. So, in order to continue the suppression of the diseases caused by this bacterium (*Streptococcus pneumoniae*), a new vaccine needs to be continuously developed to cover the new emerging serotypes (strains).[12] This feels a lot like a dog chasing its own tail.

Chapter 38: Pneumococcal vaccine – The many shades of Prevnar
[1] Centers for Disease Control and Prevention. (2017, December 6). *Pneumococcal Vaccination: What Everyone Should Know.* Retrieved from www.cdc.gov/vaccines/vpd/pneumo/public/index.html
[2] Ibid.
[3] Mount Sinai Hospital. Department of Microbiology. (n.d.). *What is Streptococcus pneumoniae or pneumococcus?.* Retrieved from www.eportal.mountsinai.ca/Microbiology/faq/pneumofaq.shtml
[4] Ibid.
[5] Ibid.
[6] Pfizer. (2016, November 16). *National Advisory Committee on Immunization (Naci) Gives Prevnar® 13 Grade a Recommendation.* Retrieved from www.pfizer.ca/national-advisory-committee-immunization-naci-gives-prevnar%C2%AE-13-grade-recommendation
[7] Pfizer. (n.d.). *Vaccines.* [2016 Annual Review]. Retrieved from www.pfizer.com/files/investors/financial_reports/annual_reports/2016/scientific-innovation/vaccines/index.html
[8] Ibid.
[9] Ibid.
[10] Pichichero, M.E. and Cary, J.R. (2007). Emergence of a multiresistant serotype 19A pneumococcal strain not included in the 7-valent conjugate vaccine as an otopathogen in children. *JAMA*, 298(15), 1772-1778
[11] Ibid.
[12] Tan T. Q. (2012). Pediatric invasive pneumococcal disease in the United States in the era of pneumococcal conjugate vaccines. *Clinical microbiology reviews*, 25(3), 409-419.

CHAPTER 39

MMR, the viral riot

*"Love is like the measles; we all have to go
through it."*

~ *Jerome K. Jerome (English writer and
humorist)*

Measles, mumps and rubella viruses cause acute infections that are dependent on humans for survival and replication.

The measles virus enters your body as you inhale. When inhaled through the respiratory tract it multiplies silently in the tissues for a week then goes into the lymph nodes and eventually enters the bloodstream. The body fights hard to produce antibodies and once it overcomes the illness, you are immune for life.

Some people say measles is a deadly disease. Perhaps it is if you live in poverty and have poor nutrition, poor sanitation and a contaminated water supply. In that case, any germ can be deadly. As long as you live under clean conditions, measles should not be a virus of much concern.

Measles virus has the ability to suppress the immune system and it's common to get secondary infections like ear infection. These secondary infections are usually treated successfully with antibiotics.

As with measles, the mumps virus is one of those viruses best contracted during childhood. When adult men get mumps, it can cause orchitis, which is an inflammation of the testicles and has been associated with infertility.

Rubella is normally a rather mild disease. It has been considered a typical childhood disease throughout history, but turns into a very serious disease for a pregnant woman when she becomes infected. If the virus spreads to the fetus, it can cause a spontaneous abortion and severely disturb the fetal developmental process which is known as congenital rubella syndrome (CRS).

A large study conducted in Japan discovered that those who had measles and mumps during childhood were significantly less likely to die from heart attacks and strokes later in life.[1] Another study showed that for each additional childhood illness, such as measles, mumps or rubella, the less likely the person was to suffer acute coronary events.[2]

The first defenders

As you may remember, our innate immune system (first responders) does not work with antibodies. It works mostly with something called natural killer (NK) cells and is often vitamin D dependent. Our innate immunity is the most important immune defense we have.

We know that people with antibodies to specific diseases may still succumb to those diseases. We also know when you have a community-acquired infection, such as measles or mumps, it engages both sides of the immune system. The Th2 cells create the antibodies and the Th1 cells are defined by knowing the difference between you and foreign substances that are not a part of you. It is also known that certain viruses, such as the measles virus, powerfully suppress immunity.[3]

A study done in Faroe Islands showed that once somebody became sick with the measles, they stayed immune to that disease for 75 years. Those who were vaccinated against measles only had immunity lasting for about 20 years. This means if vaccinated in childhood, a woman is unlikely to pass the immunity on to her baby or at least pass it on as effectively as she would have had she contracted measles naturally.

It's essential for our immune system to develop and grow by facing natural infectious challenges.

If the body is deprived of the opportunity to fight natural infections, the immune system won't gain the required strength or knowledge to fight on its own. As a consequence, a range of hidden conditions that adversely affect your immunity may be expressed. These conditions are sometimes called Th2 dominant disorders. This happens when our immune system is not challenged by normal infections or bacteria in the environment.

Our body's microbiome is primarily bacteria, viruses, and fungi. We need these naturally acquired infections to help stimulate our immune system so our body as a whole becomes stronger and keeps us healthy.

The vaccine kitchen

When preparing the chicken embryo agar to grow the viruses, scientists first incubate chicken eggs for 16 hours. (An agar being a natural gelatinous substance used in biological culture media). The shell is then cracked and the albumin removed. An albumin-saline solution is transferred to a Falcon culture dish[4].

In the MMRII[5] vaccine, the measles and mumps virus are propagated in chicken embryo,

while Rubella virus is propagated in WI-38. After these have been propagated separately, they are then combined into one vaccine. The final product will therefore not only have all three viruses, but also chicken embryo proteins from two separate cultures and human proteins. The ProQuad vaccine has the added varicella virus, which was propagated in MRC-5 cells before being combined into one vaccine.[6]

In Japan medical authorities took the Urabe AM9 mumps vaccine and gave five million doses in a single vaccine. There were few, if any, reported cases of meningitis related to the vaccine. When they combined measles, mumps and rubella, there was a dramatic increase in the adverse reactions to the mumps virus in the vaccine, mostly in the form of meningitis.

Unsurprisingly, after that scandal the Japanese authorities took the MMR vaccine off the list of recommended vaccines.[7] Their experience was that when you combine three viruses into one, you've got major problems.

The same thing happened in Bulgaria where they used a mumps strain called Sofia 6. The strain appeared to be triggering cases of meningitis, so it was discontinued.[8]

According to the *History of Vaccines* website, Stanley Plotkin, a scientist who invented the rubella vaccine, grew the rubella virus he had isolated in WI-38 cells that were kept at 86°F (30°C). Plotkin did this to force the virus to adjust to the warm temperature so that it would grow very poorly at normal body temperature. He grew the virus "through the cells 25 times" and after that, "it was no longer able to replicate enough to cause illness in a living person." It was, nonetheless, still able to provoke a protective immune response.[9]

The article then states:

> *"Rubella vaccine developed with WI-38 is still used throughout much of the world today as part of the combined MMR (measles, mumps, and rubella) vaccine."*[10]

So, in the US we have the RA273 strain, and in Japan the Takahashi strain. The Americans grew their cells on the aborted fetal cell line WI-38, and the Japanese grew theirs on a rabbit cell line.

The NIH rubella vaccine was captured from the throat of a soldier in 1961 and then grown in African green monkey kidney cells that did not harbor the SV40 virus. A Missouri-based company, Phillips-Roxanne, grew the virus in pup kidney cells, and in Belgium a company captured the virus from the urine of a sick 10-year-old girl and grew it in rabbit kidney cells.

Three vaccines were approved in 1969 and none of them used human cells. They all used animal cells and they all eventually disappeared from the market after Plotkin's vaccine was finally approved in 1979. The Philips-Roxanne vaccine only lasted six to nine months on the market because once it was used in a bigger population it was found to cause bad side-effects in kids, triggering very sore knees caused by inflammation.

A study was done to see how much aborted fetal DNA was in the vaccines. The author studied a rubella vaccine called Meruvax II, manufactured by Merck, for ssDNA and dsDNA. The average ssDNA was 142.05 ng and the average dsDNA was 35.00 ng.[11] If you recall early in this book we mention the FDA safety guidelines specify the amount of residual DNA should be *no greater than 10 ng*.

Recently, information was released that the ProQuid combination vaccine by Merck resulted in twice as many seizures when the vaccines are dispensed separately.

If guidelines are ignored, seizures can and do result.

MMR is the only vaccine that contains more than one live vaccine in one shot. This one contains three, which is why some believe the vaccine is a problem. All these viruses are swimming around together in the vial and they could interact and mutate in ways we might not have foreseen.

As mentioned above, Japan withdrew its home-produced MMR vaccine in 1993 after around 1,000 children suffered side-effects, in particular aseptic meningitis. The problem was pinned on the mumps component produced in Japan, which continued to vaccinate against measles and rubella using single vaccines.

Everyone gets vaccinated

According to WHO data, there were 16 African countries that exceeded the United States' vaccination rate of 91% for the measles-mumps-rubella vaccine in 2013.

Besides those African countries, many other parts of the world have outperformed the US in giving infants the MMR vaccine at their one-year immunization. These include Australia, China, New Zealand and most of the European countries.[12][13][14][15]

In 2017, the WHO recorded that 92% of the US population received their first dose of the measles vaccine at age one. There are countries, such as China, Cuba and Thailand that achieved as much as 99% coverage dispensing first measles vaccine dosages.

There is now no country in the world that offers single vaccines in preference to MMR. Therefore, the measles vaccine can be considered to be a three-in-one measles-mumps-rubella vaccine (and not just a measles vaccine).

Autism

The MMR vaccine has been notoriously and infamously correlated with autism, the early childhood mental condition that is increasing so drastically the Autism Society of America considers it (autism) an epidemic.

To be more specific, this correlation between the MMR vaccine and autism is linked with the measles component of the MMR vaccine. One study showed:

> *"[...] over 90% of MMR antibody-positive autistic sera were also positive for MBP autoantibodies, suggesting a strong association between MMR and CNS autoimmunity in autism."*[16]

This is saying that over 90% of the blood samples in the study had antibodies from the MMR vaccine and also autoantibodies for myelin basic protein (MBP). This protein is found in the myelin sheath covering our nerves. When a person suffers from a disease that destroys the myelin sheath, MBP can be found in the blood.[17]

When you take three live viruses and inject them into a child in a way human evolution has never seen before, the game changes and all bets are off. The outcome is simply unknown.

Viruses have been known to attack our nerves. An example of such a viral attack would be shingles. So, it should be of no surprise that when a variety of ingredients in a vaccine known to affect the nervous system is combined with three living viruses, they have the ability to destroy not only the nerves themselves, but also destroy their means of travel throughout the body.

More on the MMR vaccine and autism in the following chapter.

Chapter 39: MMR, the viral riot

[1] Kubota, Y., Iso, H., Tamakoshi, A., and JACC Study Group. (2015). Association of measles and mumps with cardiovascular disease: The Japan Collaborative Cohort (JACC) study. *Atherosclerosis*, 241(2), 682-686.

[2] Pesonen, E., Andsberg, E., Ohlin, H., Puolakkainen, M., Rautelin, H., Sama, S., and Persson, K. (2007). Dual role of infections as risk factors for coronary heart disease. *Atherosclerosis*, 192(2), 370-375

[3] Kerdile, Y.M., Sellin, C.I., Druelle, J., and Horvat, B. (2006). Immunosuppression by measles virus: role of viral proteins. *Rev Med Virol*, 16(1), 49-63

[4] Corning. (2007). *Falcon Product Selection Guide*. Retrieved from www.corning.com/media/worldwide/cls/documents/selection-guides/CLS-F-PSG-001%20REV2.pdf

[5] World Health Organization (WHO). (n.d.). *M-M-R II*. Retrieved from www.who.int/immunization_standards/vaccine_quality/PQ_168_MMR_MSD_PI_July2008.pdf

[6] Food and Drug Administration (FDA). (n.d.). *ProQuad*. Retrieved from www.fda.gov/downloads/biologicsbloodvaccines/vaccines/approvedproducts/ucm123796.pdf

[7] Tanaka, Y., Ueda, Y., Yoshino, K., & Kimura, T. (2017). History repeats itself in Japan: Failure to learn from rubella epidemic leads to failure to provide the HPV vaccine. *Human vaccines & immunotherapeutics*, 13(8), 1859-1860.

[8] Odisseev, H.1. and Gacheva, N. (1994). Vaccinoprophylaxis of mumps using mumps vaccine, strain Sofia 6, in Bulgaria. *Vaccine*, 12(14), 1251-1254

[9] The College of Physicians of Philadelphia. (2018, January 19). *Human Cell Strains in Vaccine Development*, Retrieved from www.historyofvaccines.org/content/articles/human-cell-strains-vaccine-development

[10] Ibid.

[11] Deisher, T.A., Doan, N.V., Koyama, K., and Bwabye, S. (2015). Epidemiologic and Molecular Relationship Between Vaccine Manufacture and Autism Spectrum Disorder Prevalence. *Issues Law Med*, 30(1), 47-70.

[12] The World Bank. (2018). *Countries and Economies*. Retrieved from www.data.worldbank.org/country

[13] World Health Organization (WHO). (2018, July 19). *Global Health Observatory data repository*. Retrieved from www.apps.who.int/gho/data/node.main.A826

[14] The Washingtom Post. (2015, February 3). *Map: 113 countries have higher measles immunization rates than the U.S. for 1-year-olds*. Retrieved from www.washingtonpost.com/news/worldviews/wp/2015/02/03/map-113-countries-have-higher-measles-immunization-rates-than-the-u-s-for-1-year-olds/?noredirect=on&utm_term=.b3085a84b682

[15] www.npr.org/sections/goatsandsoda/2015/02/06/384068229/measles-vaccination-rates-tanzania-does-better-than-u-s

[16] Singh, V.K., Lin, S.X., Newell, E., and Nelson, C. (2002) Abnormal measles-mumps-rubella antibodies and CNS autoimmunity in children with autism. *J Biomed Sci*, 9(4), 359-364.

[17] Mondello, S. and Hayes, R. (2015). Chapter 16 –Biomarkers. *Traumatic Brain Injury* [Vol.1, Part 1, pp. 245-265]. Waltham, MA: Elsevier B.V

CHAPTER 40

MMR—Autism and a ravaged immune system

*"A further sign of health is that we don't
become undone by fear and trembling, but we
take it as a message that it's time to stop
struggling and look directly at what's
threatening us."*

~ **Pema Chödrön** *(The Places that Scare
You)*

The FDA warns that all drugs containing human albumin could result in
prion or viral disease contamination.[1] It's worth noting the MMR vaccines
contain genetically engineered human albumin.

In 2011, Dr. Helen Ratajczak, the President of Edmond Enterprises
LLC and *Professional of the Year for 2018 in Healthcare Therapy*, looked into
some concerns over injecting human DNA into another human and how
that relates to autism.[2] In the paper, she highlights that the thimerosal-
free MMR II vaccine entered the market in 1979, but it wasn't until 1983
it became the only available vaccine.

DR. Helen Ratajczak comments:

> *"Autism in the United States spiked dramatically between
> 1983 and 1990 from 4–5/10,000 to 1/500. In 1988, two
> doses of MMR II were recommended to immunize those
> individuals who did not respond to the first injection. A
> spike of incidence of autism accompanied the addition of
> the second dose of MMR II."[3]*

She goes on to say how this MMR II vaccine was introduced in Britain
in 1988.

She continues:

> *"[...] United Kingdom, which reported a dramatic increase in prevalence of autism to 1/64 [...]. [...]. It is important to note that unlike the former MMR, the rubella component of MMR II was propagated in a human cell line derived from embryonic lung tissue (Merck and Co., Inc., 2010)."* [4]

Sugar, sugar

It has been suggested the MMR II vaccine has the ability to trigger type 1 diabetes. Several studies have been published on this matter. One suggestion, which we found interesting, is not a peer-reviewed study, but a technical report on *ResearchGate* [5]. On the author's homepage his dedication to further research into the topic is evident. [6]

The report notes that besides the measles, mumps and rubella live viruses, the major proteins in the vaccine come from the chicken embryo cell culture. It also notes a high correlation between the chicken culture proteins in the vaccine and type 1 diabetes.

How can this be?

Both animal and human cells carry a protein called glutamate decarboxylase (GAD). This is a protein associated with type 1 diabetes. The chicken proteins in the MMR II vaccine have been shown to create antibodies against GAD65 and GAD67 in chickens. Chicken and human GAD65 are 95% identical. The chicken GAD65 have then been shown to cross-react with human GAD65, which causes type 1 diabetes. (The numbers (65 and 67) depict the molecular mass of the protein). Because this report wasn't a published research paper, we studied the references used in it and found they appeared to be from reliable sources.

As many of you may know, diabetes is directly related to beta cells produced in our pancreas.

One paper the author refers to in the above report concludes:

> *"The identification of β-cell proteins as autoantigens was perhaps the defining moment for type 1 diabetes as a disease, because it represented the first evidence that placed the disease in the pathogenetic category of autoimmunity."*[7]

So, the vaccine may not contain aluminum or mercury, but it appears to have so many other ingredients it doesn't need the *help* of either of these metals to trigger serious effects in infants or children.

If not mercury or aluminum...

Perhaps the most concerning known contaminant in the MMR II vaccine is glutamate, and MMR II seems to have a lot of it. Other ingredients include live viruses grown on culture that contains gelatin. As you may recall from a chapter in Part One of this book, gelatin is made from the bones and ligaments of farm animals.

In addition to its damaging effect on the shikimate pathway, glyphosate has other *qualities* that may potentially bring with it contaminants into the vaccine that are completely unforeseen and most likely their presence never tested for.

In 2017, scientists tested various vaccines for particles that were not intended ever to be in the vaccines.[8] They tested three different MMR vaccines as detailed below.

Priorix manufactured by GlaxoSmithKline (GSK), of Italy. Among the particles found were tungsten, nickel and iron.

M-M-R vaxPro, manufactured by Sanofi Pasteur MSD, of France. Some of the particles found were stainless steel, platinum, silver, bismuth, iron and chromium.

Morupar, manufactured by what is known today as Novartis, in Italy, was the last MMR vaccine they tested. No particles were found in this vaccine.

An explanation for the presence of these metals could be the fact that glyphosate is very efficient at extracting metals. So, during the manufacturing stage if any of the equipment contain these types of particles, it's highly likely the glyphosate may drag them along into the vaccine. It's important to note here that the MMR II vaccine was not part of their study. We don't know which particles, or if any, it contains.

Back to autism

Let's return to the elephant in the room: the infamous *autism* tag associated with the measles portion of the MMR vaccine.

Can it be scientifically explained?

As we now know, the measles virus has the protein hemagglutinin on its surface. This is the part of the virus that's used in the vaccine, which means our body will create antibodies against it.

As mentioned earlier, autoimmunity can result from foreign particles being so similar to our own, that the body thinks its own proteins are the enemy. This is the case with hemagglutinin, which looks a lot like our myelin basic protein (MBP). We need this protein in order to make myelin sheath. When we're exposed to the measles protein (hemagglutinin), our body reacts the way the vaccine was designed: we make antibodies to it. A problem occurs when our body fails to see the difference between the hemagglutinin and our myelin basic protein, so in addition to attacking the invading virus, our antibodies now also start attacking our own proteins. This occurrence has been linked to autism.[9]

In the study referenced above, the scientists studied abnormal antibodies in autistic children. In their study, they tested the blood in 125 autistic children and 92 control children (not autistic children) for antibodies. Out of the 125 children with autism, in 75 of them, or 60%, the researcher found a specific MMR antibody. This specific antibody, the authors explain, "is unique to the measles subunit of the vaccine."[10]

They then tested the blood that was MMR antibody positive for MBP autoantibodies. It turned out that 90% of the samples "were also positive for MBP autoantibodies, suggesting a strong association between MMR and CNS autoimmunity in autism."[11]

Here, once again, we can see how molecular mimicry works on our immune system.

One of the authors of the above paper, neuroimmunologist Dr. Vijendra K. Singh[12], has studied this subject for quite some time. He suggests that autism could be triggered by a virus causing the body to attack its own myelin sheath.

In a 2009 paper, Dr. Singh explains:

> *"Many autistic children harbored brain myelin basic protein autoantibodies and elevated levels of antibodies to measles virus and measles-mumps-rubella (MMR) vaccine."*[13]

The author explains that the autistic children also had elevated markers for systemic inflammation, which is the same as chronic inflammation.

When we looked closer into whether vaccines cause chronic inflammation, we uncovered numerous papers rejecting any such suggestion. Among those many papers was one from 2003 by Dr. Paul Offit regarding studies that claim:

> *"Consistent with critical differences between natural infection and immunization, well-controlled epidemiologic studies do not support the hypothesis that vaccines cause autoimmunity."*[14]

An observational study was done in Yokohama, Japan. The authors used data from Kohoku Ward spanning all cases of autism spectrum disorder (ASD) that fitted within ICD-10 guidelines for children up to seven years old, born in the period from 1988 to 1996.

The authors conclude:

> *"The significance of this finding is that MMR vaccination is most unlikely to be a main cause of ASD, that it cannot explain the rise over time in the incidence of ASD, and that withdrawal of MMR in countries where it is still being used cannot be expected to lead to a reduction in the incidence of ASD."*[15]

What we found very interesting was the major rise in autism for those born in 1994. Even when considering the number of births each year, it doesn't explain the skyrocketing rise in autism for those born that year.

We looked to see if the paper mentions any changes during 1994. The only change mentioned that could account for this, is a change in vaccine schedule. But then for those born in 1995 and 1996, the numbers dropped.

Considering the drop in total births in that two-year period, this could account for the fact that in November 1994, Yokohama's city boundaries were changed and the city, on paper at least, became smaller. The authors didn't believe this made a significant difference and continued the study using the new boundaries.[16] They didn't show what the result would have been had they continued using the original boundaries.

Vaccine friendly

Dr. Paul Thomas, author of the book *The Vaccine Friendly Plan*[17] created his own vaccine schedule for his medical practice.[18] In his revised vaccine schedule, he waits until the child is three years old before giving the MMR vaccine. In 2015, Dr. Thomas attended the public hearing in Oregon on Bill SB 442, which "seeks to remove all philosophical and religious exemptions to vaccines in the State of Oregon."[19]

The article says that during this hearing, Dr. Thomas states that:

> *"[...] he does not give every vaccine to every child in his practice, and as a result, he has over 1000 children in his practice over the age of 3, and NONE of them have autism. The rest of the country is seeing a rate of about one out of 50 children on the autism spectrum."*[20]

Regardless of whether this means the MMR is linked to autism or not, if his statement is correct then we cannot help but think there must be some type of correlation between age, number of vaccines given and autism.

Dr. Thomas is not the only doctor who believes in staggering vaccines. Many healthcare professionals in the US are vaccinating their children on a schedule in which some vaccines are omitted while others are staggered. These schedules are not publicly acknowledged, but we must wonder what has caused these healthcare professionals to opt for a less aggressive vaccine schedule for their own children.

If the current official vaccine schedule is truly the best for our children, we wonder why the schedule differs from one country to another and why healthcare professionals sometimes choose their own vaccine schedule. How are we supposed to know which guidelines are best suited? Surely the concerns for childhood illnesses are similar regardless of which country you live in.

Career suicide

It's difficult to find researchers willing to put their names on papers showing any correlation between vaccines and adverse events.

There seems to be an overriding fear amongst medical professionals that suggesting vaccines trigger chronic disorders will lead to defamation or discreditation. This cautious approach, we feel, is very biased in itself, as it will discourage researchers from publishing their data or even doing the research to begin with.

(To avoid being discredited, or *supposedly* discredited, we have done our best to focus on authors and medical professionals with peer-reviewed or otherwise scientifically-accepted papers, studies and articles).

And here's another bias, the so-called Healthy User Bias (HUB). This bias covers issues such as when children prone to illnesses are not given the vaccines during safety trials. Therefore, these trials don't represent the true population receiving the vaccines.

Just because health professionals and researchers have been *defamed* or publicly ridiculed, doesn't mean they're wrong. Most of them are highly educated, but take a more holistic and natural approach to medicine.

The views of these professionals seem to be in sync with the research we have shared with you in this book. Namely, that the antibodies our bodies create to fight foreign substances can become autoantibodies and attack the body's own tissues, and also lead to chronic diseases. Diseases that are often worse than the infectious diseases they protect us from.

One of those illnesses can in some instances be a neurologic disease called subacute sclerosing panencephalitis (SSPE). This is a rare, chronic, progressive encephalitis that almost always ends in death. In fact, today, this disease is considered to be "a rare, slow viral infection caused by a defective measles virus."[21]

As with many other vaccine-related concerns, it's difficult to find published papers on this matter. The best approach seems to be to source research *unrelated* to vaccines and study the ingredients in the vaccines. Not an ideal approach—and don't we know it! It requires many hours extra reading.

Chapter 40: MMR – Autism and a ravaged immune system
[1] Cell Culture DISH. (2012, June13). *FDA Issues Guidance for Warning Labels on All Drugs Produced Using Blood Products including Plasma-derived Albumin.* Retrieved from www.cellculturedish.com/fda-issues-guidance-for-warning-labels-on-all-drugs-produced-using-blood-products-including-plasma-derived-albumin/
[2] Ratajczak, H.V. (2010). Theoretical aspects of autism: Causes—A review. *Journal of Immunotoxicology,* 8(1), 68-79
[3] Ibid.
[4] Ibid.
[5] Arumugham, V. (2017). *Role of MMR II vaccine contamination with GAD65 containing chick embryo cell culture in the etiology of type 1 diabetes.* [Technical Report]. DOI: 10.5281/zenodo.1034770
[6] ResearchGate. (n.d.). Vinu Arumugham. Retrieved from www.researchgate.net/profile/Vinu_Arumugham2
[7] Roep, B. O., & Peakman, M. (2012). Antigen targets of type 1 diabetes autoimmunity. Cold Spring Harbor perspectives in medicine, 2(4), a007781.
[8] Gatti, A.M. and Montanari, S. (2016). New Quality-Control Investigations on Vaccines: Micro- and Nanocontamination. *Int J Vaccines Vaccin,* 4(1): 00072.
[9] Singh, V.K., Lin, S.X., Newell, E., and Nelson, C. (2002) Abnormal measles-mumps-rubella antibodies and CNS autoimmunity in children with autism. *J Biomed Sci,* 9(4), 359-364.
[10] Ibid.
[11] Ibid.
[12] Wikipedia. (2018, October 6). *Vijendra K. Singh.* Retrieved from www.en.wikipedia.org/wiki/Vijendra_K._Singh
[13] Singh, V.K. (2009). Phenotypic expression of autoimmune autistic disorder (AAD): a major subset of autism. *Ann Clin Psychiatry,* 21(3), 148-161.
[14] Offit, P.A. and Hackett, C.J. (2003). Addressing Parents' Concerns: Do Vaccines Cause Allergic or Autoimmune Diseases?. *Pediatrics,* 111(3), 653-659
[15] Honda, H., Shimizu, Y., and Rutter, M. (2005) No effect of MMR withdrawal on the incidence of autism: a total population study. *J Child Psychol Psychiatry,* 46(6), 572-579.
[16] Ibid.
[17] Thomas, P. and Margulis, J. (2016). *The Vaccine-Friendly Plan: Dr. Paul's Safe and Effective Approach to Immunity and Health-from Pregnancy Through Your Child's Teen Years.* New York, N.Y: Ballantine books
[18] Dr. Paul Approved. (n.d.). *The Dr. Paul Approved Vaccine Plan.* Retrieved from www.drpaulapproved.com/uploads/6/4/8/3/64831775/dr_paul_approved_vacci ne_plan.pdf
[19] Global Research. (2015, February 25). *Vaccines Linked to Autism – Preserve Medical Freedom: Dr. Paul Thomas, M.D..* Retrieved from www.globalresearch.ca/vaccines-linked-to-autism-preserve-medical-freedom-dr-paul-thomas-m-d/5433505
[20] Ibid.

[21] Yilmaz, D., Aydin, O.F., Senbil, N., and Yuksel, D. (2006). Subacute sclerosing panencephalitis: Is there something different in the younger children? *Brain and Development*, 28(10), 649-652

CHAPTER 41

Varicella—The chicken itch

"Varicella always runs a favourable course.
It has no sequelae."

~ Alex. Collie (Dictionary of Medicine
1894, p. 318)

You may recall comments on immunoglobulins and how IgA is most abundant in the mucosal tissues. There's IgA in smaller amounts in the serum, but we can tell the difference because secretory immunoglobulin A (sIgA) always comes in pairs (dimer). Our mucosal tissues are a part of our innate immune system. You may also recall that this is our first line of defense and the part of our immune system vaccines bypass completely.

This is important for newborns because as we have now established a vaccine does not trigger the production of the antibody sIgA. Although all types of immunoglobulins are found in the human breast milk, more than 90% of them are sIgA.[1] This is unfortunate for newborns if they are being breastfed by a mother who has received her antibodies through vaccinations rather than natural occurring infections.

Let's put this into a perspective. Varicella-zoster aka chickenpox is a childhood illness most adults today recall going through. It consisted usually of a week in bed feeling miserable. The trade-off being lifelong immunity.

Today's children are being vaccinated and don't have to go through this week-long misery. As a trade-off, they don't get lifelong immunity. Instead, they either risk contracting chickenpox later in life or they are at a higher risk of contracting shingles. The elderly aren't being indirectly immunized anymore by being exposed to children with chickenpox. This means they have lost their natural immunity boosts against shingles in their old age.

Shingles is a varicella-zoster virus at work.[2] When a person contracts chickenpox a second time, it's referred to as *shingles*. This time the virus travels to the spinal cord and affects the nerves. It's very painful, resulting in blisters in a specific area of your body, usually around the trunk or face.

Research has shown that cases of shingles, in children as in adults, have become more prevalent with the increased use of varicella vaccinations.[34]

What has the vaccine industry done to solve this unfortunate rise in herpes-zoster infection? They created a shingles vaccine. This vaccine is given to adults only, so we aren't including it in this book.

Perhaps it won't surprise you to learn that the shingles vaccine is manufactured by the same company that manufactures the varicella vaccine. The varicella virus only grows well in human cells and tends to only infect humans. For the production of the varicella vaccine therefore, it needs human cells for growth and replication.

In the making

Merck's Varivax vaccine used today originated from the Japanese Oka vaccine strain. It was originally collected from a child infected with a wild varicella infection. The virus was grown in human cell culture and then propagated in embryonic guinea pig cell culture and WI-38 human cell culture. When the virus reached Merck Research Laboratories (MRL), their laboratory grew the virus in MRC-5 human diploid cell cultures.

The vaccine may not contain aluminum or thimerosal, but it does include gelatin, MSG and neomycin in addition to the human and animal cells.

Immunocompromised

Several neurological disorders have been associated with the varicella vaccine. When a child who receives the chickenpox vaccine grows older and their immunity wanes, they become infected with the virus as an adult. The disease is now much more severe than if they had caught it as a child. They are now at a high risk of developing secondary problems like pneumonia and other infections.

Merck's vaccine Varivax warns in its package insert not to give the vaccine to immunocompromised individuals:

> *"VARIVAX is a live, attenuated varicella-zoster vaccine (VZV) and may cause an extensive vaccine-associated rash or disseminated disease in individuals who are immunosuppressed or immunodeficient."*[5]

Merck doesn't stop there, they continue warning that even:

> *"[...] in patients with a family history of congenital or hereditary immunodeficiency until the patient's immune status has been evaluated and the patient has been found to be immunocompetent."*[6]

Throughout the package insert, they stress concerns and warn against effects related to the wild-caught chickenpox illness. We wonder if doctors are aware of this and, if they are, whether they highlight some of these concerns to the parents.

One such concern would be:

> *"Avoid use of salicylates (aspirin) or salicylate-containing products in children and adolescents 12 months through 17 years of age for six weeks following vaccination with VARIVAX because of the association of Reye syndrome with aspirin therapy and wild-type varicella infection."*[7]

Regardless of the various DNA from humans and animals, and other ingredients which are of concern, we were unable to find specific immune or neurological illnesses tied to the chickenpox vaccine. Most articles and papers highlight the correlation between the vaccine and the growing incidences of shingles.

If there's a reason to be concerned about human and animal DNA causing problems in other vaccines then surely there would be issues with it in this one as well?

We have a couple of thoughts on how to answer this question—one of them relating to the warnings in the package insert. Because of this concern, physicians are very careful not to vaccinate the immunocompromised children or children with immunocompromised family members. Children vaccinated with this vaccine are going to be the children in good health.

The other thought is that as this vaccine is not given until 12 months of age and is simultaneously administered with HepA, MMR, (influenza), IPV, PCV13, Hib, DTaP and HepB vaccines, it's possible the side-effects of the chickenpox vaccine are recorded as side-effects for one of the other (listed) vaccines.

Chapter 41: Varicella – The chicken itch

[1] Ballabio, C., Bertino, E., Coscia, A., Fabris, C., Fuggetta, D., Molfino., … Restani, P. (2007). Immunoglobulin-A Profile in Breast Milk From Mothers Delivering Full Term and Preterm Infants. *International Journal of Immunopathology and Pharmacology*, 20(1), 119-128

[2] Mayo Clinic. (2018, May 16). *Shingles*. Retrieved from www.mayoclinic.org/diseases-conditions/shingles/symptoms-causes/syc-20353054

[3] Edmunds, W.J. and Brisson, M. (2002). The effect of vaccination on the epidemiology of varicella zoster virus. *J Infect*, 44(4), 211-219.

[4] Cision PR Web. (2003, October 2). *DATA REVEALS THREAT OF SHINGLES EPIDEMIC FROM VACCINE USE Health Officials Threaten Legal Action Against Researcher*. Retrieved from www.prweb.com/releases/2003/10/prweb82645.htm

[5] Merck. (2018, October). *Varivax*. Retrieved from www.merck.com/product/usa/pi_circulars/v/varivax/varivax_pi.pdf

[6] Ibid.

[7] Ibid.

CHAPTER 42

Rotavirus—The runs

*"When health is absent, wisdom cannot
reveal itself, art cannot manifest, strength
cannot fight, wealth becomes useless, and
intelligence cannot be applied."*

~ **Herophilus** *(Greek physician)*

Rotavirus causes severe diarrhea. Unless you don't have access to hospital care, even the most severe case is normally not a huge concern. This is because the main side effect of severe diarrhea is dehydration, and in hospital it will be treated with IV fluids. In countries which lack medical care, diarrhea is a very serious illness.

A paper from the Cochrane Library in 2012 states that:

> *"Rotavirus results in more diarrhoea-related deaths in children less than five years of age than any other single agent in countries with high childhood mortality. It is also a common cause of diarrhoea-related hospital admissions in countries with low childhood mortality."*[1]

Although there may be disagreement over the need of this vaccine in areas with good healthcare, it may save lives in other areas of the world.

Dr, Leonard Friedland who works for GlaxoSmithKline (GSK) said during a hearing arranged by the FDA in 2010 that:

> *"[...] rotavirus infection is the leading cause of severe diarrhea in both developed and developing countries. Prior to the development of vaccines against rotavirus, worldwide one child died from rotavirus every minute. To date, vaccination is the only effective preventative*

strategy. Its widespread use has the potential to prevent about two million deaths over the next decade."[2]

We can see how scary this disease is for people in developing countries who experience the severity of the rotavirus on a regular basis. So why the controversy towards a vaccine that is designed to save literally millions of lives?

Trials

As we have mentioned before, it seems difficult to figure out how any conclusions can be drawn from vaccine trials. We are aware of the guidelines the researchers have to follow. One of those guidelines being that it's unethical to give a salt solution as the placebo when there's an effective vaccine against the germ. Therefore, it's not surprising that the placebo is never specified as being a saline solution. It most likely isn't saline. It should never be expected that it is, unless specified.

We looked at both Rotateq[3] and Rotarix[4] study designs. Neither specifies what they used as a placebo. We are surprised this is not a requirement. The RotaTeq vaccine study design states their placebo matched that of the RotaTeq vaccine. We're not sure what that means, although it sounds like a different brand or version of rotavirus vaccine may have been used. In addition, as with so many if not most vaccine trials, the vaccines were not given alone. They were given in combination with HepB, flu, DTaP, pneumococcal and polio vaccines.[5]

As before, we have difficulty understanding how it's possible to know which events are related to each vaccine. Because these trials usually include other vaccines as well, we are not certain how the scientists know which vaccine or component to attribute a side effect to.

Is it possible a vaccine is deemed safe because its side-effects are attributed to or labeled under the wrong vaccine?

With these biases and the inherent significant errors in mind, the clinical studies reported 52 deaths:

"There were 25 deaths in the RotaTeq recipients compared to 27 deaths in the placebo recipients. The most common cause of death was sudden infant death syndrome."[6]

In regards to the Rotarix vaccine, combining observations made in eight clinical trials, the scientists reported a total of 68 deaths after vaccination with the Rotarix vaccine and 50 "deaths following placebo administration." They also observed that "[t]he most common cause of death following vaccination was pneumonia, [...]."[7]

Another serious adverse event common enough to receive special mention in package inserts for both RotaTeq and Rotarix is the ailment known as intussusception. This is an obstruction in the infants' bowels. As we mentioned, this is when the bowels more or less fold in on themselves, much like a telescope. Blood is no longer able to flow properly through the intestines and the rectum starts bleeding.

Severe combined immunodeficiency (SCID) has been associated with the rotavirus vaccine. This is when infants start out with prolonged gastroenteritis and are later diagnosed with SCID. So, in December 2009, Rotateq added SCID as a contraindication to its label.

According to Dr. David Martin, who works for the FDA, in 2010 GSK were in the middle of conducting two controlled observational studies.

Regarding these trials and referring to the Vaccine Safety Data (VSD), Dr. Martin said at that time, that:

> "[...] less than 5,000 doses have been administered. Outcomes include intussusception, seizures, meningitis/encephalitis, myocarditis, gram negative sepsis, gastrointestinal bleeding, Kawasaki disease, and hospitalized pneumonia."[8]

Vaccine manufacturers are permitted to use cell material from bodies of mammals, including humans, monkeys, cows, pigs, dogs and rodents as well as cells from birds and insects in either experimental or currently licensed vaccines. They are even experimenting with human fetal retinal cells, which have a history of causing cancerous cells in animals.

So, have other cells they use for making vaccine.

Scientists can't actually explain why the Rotarix vaccine works. They don't understand how the body's antibody production against this vaccine works or how it plays a part in protection against the actual disease. All they are sure of is that the vaccine makes its way into the small intestine and triggers an immune response.[9]

Side effects

The Rotarix and RotaTeq vaccines are made slightly different, but the rotavirus for both vaccines was derived from human cells. In addition, the RotaTeq virus was also taken from a bovine source. The rotaviruses were then propagated in Vero cells. As you may recall, Vero cells are African green monkey kidney cells which are grown in fetal bovine serum (FBS).

In 2009, a study was performed on physicians' vaccination practices. Some 25 out of 416 general practitioners said they would not vaccinate for rotavirus and 16 out of 138 subspecialists would not vaccinate for rotavirus.

Out of 70 physicians, 63 had their own children opt out of at least one of the vaccines. The reason they gave were *safety* and *too many vaccines given at once*.

The reasons given (for opting out) *specifically for the rotavirus* include:

> "*In developed countries Rotavirus is for the most part treatable and I've seen some side effects.*
>
> "*Severity of illness itself is usually not severe enough to warrant vaccination (rotavirus).*"[10]

Apart from all the ingredients purposely added to vaccines in the manufacturing stage, the rotavirus vaccines are better known for other contaminants that made their way into the vaccine.

The most infamous rotavirus vaccine contaminants have been identified as porcine circoviruses 1 and 2 (PCV1 and PCV2). We look at these in the next chapter.

Chapter 42: Rotavirus – The runs

[1] Soares-Weiser, K., Maclehose, H., Bergman, H., Ben-Aharon, I., Nagpal, S., Goldberg, E., … Cunliffe, N. (2012). Vaccines for preventing rotavirus diarrhoea: vaccines in use. *Cochrane Database of Systematic Reviews*, 11, CD008521

[2] Food and Drug Administration. and Center for Biologics Evaluation and Research. (2010, May 7). *FDA Vaccine and Related Biological Product Advisory Committee Meeting.* [Transcript].   Retrieved   from   www.wayback.archive-it.org/7993/20170405194334/https://www.fda.gov/downloads/AdvisoryCommi ttees/CommitteesMeetingMaterials/BloodVaccinesandOtherBiologics/Vaccinesa ndRelatedBiologicalProductsAdvisoryCommittee/UCM215266.pdf

[3] NIH U.S. National Library of Medicine. (2015, October 5). *Rotavirus Efficacy and Safety Trial (REST)(V260-006).* Retrieve from www.clinicaltrials.gov/ct2/show/results/NCT00090233

[4] www.clinicaltrials.gov/ct2/show/record/NCT00480324

[5] NIH U.S. National Library of Medicine. (2018, June 8). *Efficacy, Safety, Reactogenicity & Immunogenicity of the Rotarix Vaccine in Japanese Infants.* Retrieved from www.clinicaltrials.gov/ct2/show/NCT00480324

[6] Food and Drug Administration. (2017, February). *RotaTeq.* Retrieved from www.fda.gov/downloads/biologicsbloodvaccines/vaccines/approvedproducts/uc m142288.pdf

[7] Food and Drug Administration. (n.d.). *Rotarix.* Retrieved from www.fda.gov/downloads/biologicsbloodvaccines/vaccines/approvedproducts/uc m133539.pdf

[8] Food and Drug Administration. and Center for Biologics Evaluation and Research. (2010, May 7). *FDA Vaccine and Related Biological Product Advisory Committee Meeting.* [Transcript. p. 15]. Retrieved from www.wayback.archive-it.org/7993/20170405194334/https://www.fda.gov/downloads/AdvisoryCommi ttees/CommitteesMeetingMaterials/BloodVaccinesandOtherBiologics/Vaccinesa ndRelatedBiologicalProductsAdvisoryCommittee/UCM215266.pdf

[9] Food and Drug Administration. (n.d.). *Rotarix.* Retrieved from www.fda.gov/downloads/biologicsbloodvaccines/vaccines/approvedproducts/uc m133539.pdf

[10] Martin, M. and Badalyan, V. (2012). Vaccination practices among physicians and their children. *Open Journal of Pediatrics*, 2, 228-235.

CHAPTER 43

Rotavirus—and the porcine invaders

"We can't predict what a virus we've never seen will do."

*~ **Marc Lipsitch** (Professor of Epidemiology)*

Many uninvited guests, or as scientists would call them, *adventitious agents,* find their way into the vaccine manufacturing process. These agents fall into many categories, including bacteria, mycoplasma, parasites and viruses. The PCV1 and PCV2 viruses were uninvited agents that were discovered in the rotavirus vaccines.

In the manufacturing process for Rotarix and RotaTeq, DNA from PCV1 was detected. In the RotaTeq, PCV1 and PCV2 were detected. This was even acknowledged in their package inserts.

Multiple studies can be found online that indicate that PCV1 is harmless in pigs and PCV2 is pathogenic in pigs, but there is no evidence of either causing harm to humans. Therefore, the manufacturers have not seen a reason to remove these particles from vaccines.

That said, it's interesting to note the FDA expresses safety concerns yet allows unintended viruses, which they can't guarantee won't mutate, remain in the vaccines. As a matter of fact, the National Vaccine Information Center (NVIC), together with Dr. Joseph Mercola[1] fought to take RotaTeq (Merck) vaccine off the market. They said the vaccine was "contaminated with parts of a lethal virus that infects pigs—porcine circovirus 2 (PCV2)"[2] and wanted Merck to "publicly pledge to clean-up the vaccine."[3]

On May 7th, 2010, GSK, producer of the Rotarix vaccine, admitted their vaccine was infected with the non-lethal virus PCV1. They also "publicly pledged to re-formulate the rotavirus vaccine"[4]. GSK ended up removing the PCV1 from their vaccines. *Merck did not follow suit.*

There seems to be more concern over the RotaTeq (Merck) vaccine as it's the one that contains the PCV2 virus.

The NVIC website continues by explaining how in the end, the FDA decided to revoke their "suspension of Rotarix vaccine recommendation and" deem both Rotarix and RotaTeq vaccines safe. They did this knowing that both vaccines "remain contaminated and safety data on PCV2 contamination of RotaTeq was not evaluated by the FDA advisory committee."[5]

Circoviruses such as PCV are the smallest viruses we know of. The filters used for viruses in vaccine manufacturing are not known to protect against them as the PCV particles are too small. Regular inactivation methods do not work on PCVs.

There are multiple biological products being used in the manufacturing of vaccines. Many of these are a source of viral contaminants. We have, for instance, blood and trypsin that are taken from a common source and used in multiple vaccines. This has prompted investigations to see whether PCV1 is present in the stocks of these materials.

The polio vaccine (IPV) manufactured by GSK uses the same master Vero cell bank as the Rotarix vaccine does. They tested the beginning phases of the manufacturing process of IPV and the final product. PCV1 was found in the beginning phases, but by the time they had finished the process, the vaccine tested negative for the PCV1 virus.

After much investigation, both PCV1 and PCV2 were said to be safe for humans. Not everyone agrees with these findings. It was a big enough concern that in 2010 the advisory committee held a hearing to discuss the matter.

In this 2010 hearing, Dr. Barbara Howe, Vice President and Director of North American Vaccine Development for GSK at the time stated:

> *"It is known that PCV1 causes widespread infection in pigs. For example, about 60–95 percent of pigs tested in Germany and 26 to 55 percent of pigs tested in Canada are positive for PCV1 antibodies."[6]*

Dr. Howe shares observations found in other studies and continues:

> *"Therefore, the available data indicates that the PCV1 is not pathogenic. In fact, the non-pathogenic virus, the PCV1 is used as a vaccine vector in the first USDA fully-licensed kill vaccine against PCV2."*[7]

The vaccine manufacturers were questioned about the circovirus contaminations in their vaccines and a couple of specific research studies were used as examples. However, there is no reference to them in the transcript. We only know them by the names of their authors, *the Hattermann study and the Li study.*

When looking for the presence of PCV, *the Li study* only tested the antibodies in the blood. In *the Hattermann study,* they used samples of blood, urine and lymph nodes to look for DNA. Neither study used stool samples to look for viral DNA.

Dr. Andrew Cheung[8] who at the time, worked for the USDA Agriculture Research Service in Ames, Iowa, referred to a study performed in Canada. In this study they observed the two viruses, PCV1 and PCV2, recombine.[9]

As far as we know, there have not been any studies done on how immunosuppressed pigs or immunosuppressed humans would react if infected with PCV1.

The porcine circovirus expert, Dr. X.J Meng[10], a professor of Molecular Virology at the College of Veterinary Medicine, Virginia Tech., has been studying this virus since 1999. Dr. Meng states that an infectious clone of PCV1 exists in pigs.[11]

It seems nobody is sufficiently concerned to look at human cells yet. Easier to stick to animal studies perhaps.

Dr. Emmanuel Hanon[12], Vice President of Early Research and Development for GSK, states that GSK speculates the PCV1 comes from the trypsin they used when producing their master cell bank (MCB). In order to eliminate PCV1 from the vaccines, they would have to create a new cell bank and begin a long process spanning several years. This would necessitate conducting new clinical trials for the vaccines.[13]

A Master Cell Bank (MCB) takes the cell lines produced in a lab and tests them for authenticity, viability and contamination. Then they culture them in the ideal setting for optimal growth and then store them in most appropriate way. The MCB keeps very detailed records of all information pertaining to the cells they store, encouraging manufacturing companies to return to acquire cells for their cultures.

Dr. Hanon explains how they had found a PCV1 messenger RNA (mRNA), which is a sign that the viral particle can cause disease.[14] The mRNA is a very important part of the coding process. It takes the DNA information out of the cell nucleus and carries it into the part of the cell that makes proteins.[15] So finding a viral particle containing mRNA is finding a viral particle carrying genetic information.

The vaccine manufacturer GSK doesn't seem concerned about these findings even though the infected PCV1 gene multiplies in human cells. The reason given is because that wouldn't trigger a "productive infection."

Dr. Gary Dubin, Vice President of Global Clinical Development at GSK, states:

> "[...] there is evidence of a detection of rotavirus antigen in stools in a sizeable proportion of infants for a limited period of time. It tends to be detected later, and it tends to persist for a longer period of time, which reflects, we think, the nature of the fact that the virus in the vaccine does cause limited replication in the gut, and that is part of the mechanism of action."[16]

The concerns and study trials relating to the PCV1 in Rotarix have led to an amendment in the post-marketing part of the package insert.

The following has been added:

> "[...] intussusception including death and temporal association, Kawasaki disease and rotavirus gastroenteritis in patients with severe combined immunodeficiency syndrome."[17]

One of the most intriguing statements to come from this hearing was made by a guest speaker, Dr. Gordon Allan[18] from Queen's University of Belfast. He was speaking as an expert in porcine circoviruses. Dr. Allan explained that in order to trigger a good PCV2 infection in pigs, you first infect them with the virus and then you stimulate their immune system. The immune system is stimulated by either infecting them again or by giving them a vaccine.

Dr. Allan continues:

> *"I don't know what the vaccination schedule for children is, but if you are giving them PCV1 and then giving them another vaccine, you are immuno stimulating them. I'm not saying it is dangerous. I'm just pointing out that for PCV2 in pigs, you will not get good disease unless you immunostimulate them, not immunosuppress them, immunostimulate them."*[19]

Dr. Harry Greenberg[20] with Stanford University made a good point when he suggested that it would be nice to see studies done on the effect the vaccine has on severely immunosuppressed children. He pointed out although they should not receive the vaccine, they still do, as they are not always diagnosed as immunosuppressed until after vaccination.

Another worthy suggestion was made by Dr. Pablo Sanchez[21] with University of Texas, Southwestern Medical Center, in Dallas. He wanted to know if it was possible to look for PCV in various tissues in infants who died after receiving the vaccine. For instance, the infants who die from SIDS are already being autopsied, so a large-scale study could be conducted on testing the various tissues in these infants.

There's obviously much awareness of adventitious agents, or uninvited guests, in the vaccines. Studies are being funded to look into their effects, but we can't help wonder why every aspect is not being covered given the opportunity to do so is there? It appears researchers are still using small sample sizes, only looking at healthy infants and limiting the sources they derive their samples from.

We also wonder if they considered the fact that it could take a while for a virus to replicate. Not all viruses replicate and infect at the same rate. So, when researchers say a virus replicates and doesn't cause infection in human cells, did they also look at the rate it was replicating at? What if it takes X amount of viruses before disease results, but the study did not last long enough to determine whether this were to occur? Or, while replicating in human cells, at what rate did the virus mutate? Did the mutations replicate faster or were they more invasive?

We feel some of these questions could be answered by following through with the excellent suggestions made by doctors Sanchez and Greenberg regarding how to gain a better understanding of the true effects the PCV1 & 2 has on infants.

Chapter 43: Rotavirus – and the porcine invaders

[1] Mercola. (2019, January 19). *Mercola. Take Control of Your Health.* Retrieved from https://www.mercola.com/

[2] National Vaccine Information Center. (2010, May 20). *Vaccine Safety Critics Call For RotaTeq Vaccine Recall & Clean-Up.* Retrieved from www.nvic.org/NVIC-Vaccine-News/May-2010/Vaccine-Safety-Critics-Call-For-RotaTeq-Vaccine-Re.aspx

[3] Ibid.

[4] Ibid.

[5] Ibid.

[6] *FDA Vaccine and Related Biological Product Advisory Committee Meeting.* (2010 May 7). (Testimony of Dr. Barbara Howe). [Transcript. p. 33]. Retrieved from www.wayback.archive-it.org/7993/20170405194334/ www.fda.gov/downloads/AdvisoryCommittees/CommitteesMeetingMaterials/Bl oodVaccinesandOtherBiologics/VaccinesandRelatedBiologicalProductsAdvisoryC ommittee/UCM215266.pdf

[7] *FDA Vaccine and Related Biological Product Advisory Committee Meeting.* [Transcript. pp. 33-34]. Retrieved from www.wayback.archive-it.org/7993/20170405194334/https://www.fda.gov/downloads/AdvisoryCommi ttees/CommitteesMeetingMaterials/BloodVaccinesandOtherBiologics/Vaccinesa ndRelatedBiologicalProductsAdvisoryCommittee/UCM215266.pdf

[8] Federal Pay. (n.d.). *Federal Employee Profile – Andrew K. Cheung.* Retrieved from www.federalpay.org/employees/agricultural-research-service/cheung-andrew-k

[9] *FDA Vaccine and Related Biological Product Advisory Committee Meeting.* (2010 May 7). (Testimony of Andrew K. Cheung). [Transcript. p. 39]. Retrieved from www.wayback.archive-it.org/7993/20170405194334/ www.fda.gov/downloads/AdvisoryCommittees/CommitteesMeetingMaterials/Bl oodVaccinesandOtherBiologics/VaccinesandRelatedBiologicalProductsAdvisoryC ommittee/UCM215266.pdf

[10] Virginia-Maryland College of Veterinary Medicine. (n.d.). *Biomedical Sciences & Pathology Faculty.* Retrieved from www.vetmed.vt.edu/people/bios/meng.asp

[11] *FDA Vaccine and Related Biological Product Advisory Committee Meeting.* [Transcript. p. 39]. Retrieved from www.wayback.archive-it.org/7993/20170405194334/ www.fda.gov/downloads/AdvisoryCommittees/CommitteesMeetingMaterials/Bl oodVaccinesandOtherBiologics/VaccinesandRelatedBiologicalProductsAdvisoryC ommittee/UCM215266.pdf

[12] My Bio. (n.d.). *Bio International Convention, Personal Event Planner.* Retrieved from www.mybio.org/profile/member/1122068

[13] *FDA Vaccine and Related Biological Product Advisory Committee Meeting.* (2010 May 7). (Testimony of Dr. Emmanuel Hanon). [Transcript. p. 42]. Retrieved from www.wayback.archive-it.org/7993/20170405194334/ www.fda.gov/downloads/AdvisoryCommittees/CommitteesMeetingMaterials/Bl oodVaccinesandOtherBiologics/VaccinesandRelatedBiologicalProductsAdvisoryC ommittee/UCM215266.pdf

[14] *FDA Vaccine and Related Biological Product Advisory Committee Meeting.* [Transcript. p. 44]. Retrieved from www.wayback.archive-it.org/7993/20170405194334/ www.fda.gov/downloads/AdvisoryCommittees/CommitteesMeetingMaterials/Bl oodVaccinesandOtherBiologics/VaccinesandRelatedBiologicalProductsAdvisoryC ommittee/UCM215266.pdf

[15] NIH National Human Genome Research Institute. (n.d.). *Messenger RNA (mRNA).* Retrieved from www.genome.gov/glossary/index.cfm?id=123

[16] *FDA Vaccine and Related Biological Product Advisory Committee Meeting.* (2010 May 7). (Testimony of Dr. Gary Dubin). [Transcript. p. 68]. Retrieved from www.wayback.archive-it.org/7993/20170405194334/ www.fda.gov/downloads/AdvisoryCommittees/CommitteesMeetingMaterials/Bl oodVaccinesandOtherBiologics/VaccinesandRelatedBiologicalProductsAdvisoryC ommittee/UCM215266.pdf

[17] *FDA Vaccine and Related Biological Product Advisory Committee Meeting.* [Transcript. pp. 78-79]. Retrieved from www.wayback.archive-it.org/7993/20170405194334/ www.fda.gov/downloads/AdvisoryCommittees/CommitteesMeetingMaterials/Bl oodVaccinesandOtherBiologics/VaccinesandRelatedBiologicalProductsAdvisoryC ommittee/UCM215266.pdf

[18] Queen's University Belfast. (n.d.). *Professor Gordon Allan.* Retrieved from www.pure.qub.ac.uk/portal/en/persons/gordon-allan(16bbeeec-48e7-446a-9edf-4a7119a1727a).html

[19] *FDA Vaccine and Related Biological Product Advisory Committee Meeting.* (2010 May 7). (Testimony of Dr. Gordon Allan). [Transcript. p. 112]. Retrieved from www.wayback.archive-it.org/7993/20170405194334/ www.fda.gov/downloads/AdvisoryCommittees/CommitteesMeetingMaterials/Bl oodVaccinesandOtherBiologics/VaccinesandRelatedBiologicalProductsAdvisoryC ommittee/UCM215266.pdf

[20] Stanford University. (n.d.). *Harry B Greenberg.* Retrieved from www.profiles.stanford.edu/harry-greenberg

[21] Nationwide Children's. (n.d.). *Pablo J. Sanchez.* MD. Retrieved from www.nationwidechildrens.org/find-a-doctor/profiles/pablo-j-sanchez

CHAPTER 44

The gut and the brain

"Within one linear centimeter of your lower colon there lives and works more bacteria (about 100 billion) than all humans who have ever been born. Yet many people continue to assert that it is we who are in charge of the world."

~ *Neil deGrasse Tyson (American astrophysicist)*

Within the health sector, there has been much research done on communication between our enteric nervous system (ENS) and our central nervous system (CNS). An article in *the Scientific American* talks about a recent study on the relationship between the two.

The article states that:

> *"[...] scientists were shocked to learn that about 90 percent of the fibers in the primary visceral nerve, the vagus, carry information from the gut to the brain and not the other way around."*[1]

The article continues on explaining the association between the two *brains* (the gut being the second brain) and disorders such as irritable bowel syndrome:

> *"[...] in fact 95 percent of the body's serotonin is found in the bowels. [...]. Irritable bowel syndrome – which afflicts more than two million Americans – also arises in part from too much serotonin in our entrails, and could perhaps be regarded as a 'mental illness' of the second brain."*[2]

When we hear statements like that, it's not surprising to learn that irritable bowel syndrome (IBS) has been known to plague children with autism spectrum disorder (ASD).[34] When it comes to diagnosis and how our view on the syndrome in general has evolved, the aforementioned paper states that:

> "[w]hat was once viewed as an untreatable disease solely concerning the brain is now considered a dysfunction of the central nervous system (CNS) with accompanying disorders of the body in general as well as different organs/systems such as the immunological system or digestive tract."[5]

There have also been studies that show a correlation between ASD and pathogens in the colon and intestines.[67] It may therefore not surprise you to know that children diagnosed with ASD experience positive changes in behavior when put on healthy food regimen.[89]

The brain, stress and anxiety

There have been numerous studies confirming the correlation between autoimmunity and autism spectrum disorders (ASD). As many already know, children with ASD are sensitive to foods, so it shouldn't come as a surprise that this autoimmunity often includes gluten antibodies, and milk antigens. Another antigen that may sound familiar and is a common one in this case, is the measles antigen.[101112] This antigen has also been known to affect proteins in the brains of children with ASD.[13]

Celiac disease is an autoimmune disease in which the affected person is unable to digest gluten as gluten harms the small intestine. This disease turns out to be quite similar to autism. They both show brain injury related to food allergens like gluten. There have been more than 100 studies that have found correlation between these diseases and seizures, cranial nerve damage, dementia and impaired frontal lobe function.[1415161718]

A Harvard University researcher confirmed after a 2012 study the link between autism and inflammatory bowel disease.

In a 2015 article, he is quoted saying:

> *"From these population studies, larger than any to date, we find solid and reproducible evidence that the parents were right – as usual, [...]. Based on the data I've seen, I suspect we will soon be able to define several distinct subtypes of ASD-associated bowel diseases."*[19]

The most common neurological damage in autism is located in the cerebellum. We have cells in the cerebellum called Purkinje cells. Gluten antibodies have been seen to cross-react with these cells. In the brain of an individual with autism, most of the Purkinje cells are gone.

Children diagnosed with ASD have been found to usually have either relatives with allergies or their own personal history of allergies. Normally, people with these allergies have a negative skin or RAST test. This has led some scientist to believe ASD is related to "mast cell activation by non-allergic triggers."[20][21] It has been suggested one of those triggers may be mercury.[22]

Vaccines have all types of antigens, not just from germs or toxins, but also food-related antigens. This triggers the microglia, which are cells in the brain and spinal cord, to become overstimulated.

Mast cells (MCs) can be found near neurons and microglia. They are believed to play an important role in giving molecules access to the brain. So, it comes as no surprise we have a vast number of mast cells near the blood-brain barrier (BBB).

When we are stressed, our hypothalamus secretes corticotropin-releasing factor (CRF). This factor works synergistically with neurotensin (NT), which regulates dopamine pathways. Together, they can aggravate the mast cells to the point of breaking the blood-brain barrier. Their synergistic reactions can cause the mast cells to cause brain fog and autism spectrum disorder (ASD). When the serum of children with ASD was tested, it was found to have elevated levels of both CRF and NT.[23]

In this way, by weakening the blood-brain barrier, the mast cells (MC) have been shown to take part in the development of autism.[24]

The role of corticotropin-releasing hormone (CRH) and neurotensin (NT) doesn't stop there. CRH and NT are extremely sensitive to stress, so when the body is under a lot of stress they will activate the mast cells to promote an inflammatory process. Some scientists say this contributes to Chronic Fatigue Syndrome (CFS) and fibromyalgia.[25]

This may seem farfetched, but anxiety and stress have been shown to be common in children with ME/CFS[26] and as mentioned above, CFS can trigger inflammation that can affect the brain. This begs the question, which we have not attempted to answer in this book, whether high anxiety and stress can trigger brain dysfunctions.

ASIA

Interestingly enough, all the important mediators said to trigger ME/CFS can be traced to implicate the mast cells (MC), which are the cells near, among other places, our blood-brain barrier (BBB).

A syndrome that arose as a consequence of vaccination is the autoimmune syndrome induced by adjuvants (ASIA)[2728]. ME/CFS falls under the ASIA umbrella.

Another illness that falls under this umbrella is macrophagic myofasciitis (MF or MMF). The main symptom of this disease is that the macrophages gravitate around the injection site and are filled with aluminum hydroxide from the vaccines. This is called granuloma, which is the name for a cluster of macrophages that have gathered around the injected area and caused inflammation. This is known as Macrophagic (by macrophages) Myofasciitis (inflammation of muscle tissue).

A paper published in 2013 explains how researchers injected mice with aluminum to see what would happen. They noticed that the macrophages engulfed the metal particles, forming granulomas. These granulomas then started spreading to other organs, including the brain.[29]

The reason it's so difficult to eliminate the aluminum adjuvant captured by macrophages is because when a macrophage sees a foreign substance, it *hugs* the invader and pulls it inside. Once the invader is inside the cell membrane, the macrophage tears it into multiple tiny fragments. Some individuals don't have the ability to eliminate the toxins, so instead it just accumulates inside their macrophages.

When presented with multiple vaccines simultaneously or in a short period of time, just about anybody can be the victim of overwhelmed macrophages. In most individuals, these granulomas become smaller with time and eventually disappear. But then you have the few individuals who, for some reason or other, have difficulties facilitating this process and it ends up having dire consequences.

Another disease that falls under the ASIA umbrella is the Gulf War Syndrome (GWS). You don't have to have been anywhere near Kuwait or the Persian Gulf to be diagnosed with the GWS, although it's normally isolated to those in the military since it was the anthrax vaccine that caused severe problems for military personnel in the Gulf War.

This book is focused on childhood vaccines, which does not include the anthrax vaccine, so we'll make it quick. Many believe it was the squalene in the vaccine that was causing the GWS. The squalene is used instead of gelatin as many are allergic to that animal-product. Other vaccines that use squalene are some of the influenza vaccines. It's perhaps worth noting that the anthrax vaccine contains aluminum and GWS is said to be very much like macrophagic myofasciitis (MMF).[30]

Chapter 44: The gut and the brain

[1] Scientific American. (2010, February 12). *Think Twice: How the Gut's "Second Brain" Influences Mood and Well-Being.* Retrieved from www.scientificamerican.com/article/gut-second-brain/

[2] Scientific American. (2010, February 12). *Think Twice: How the Gut's "Second Brain" Influences Mood and Well-Being.* Retrieved from www.scientificamerican.com/article/gut-second-brain/

[3] Wasilewska, J. and Klukowski, M. (2015). Gastrointestinal symptoms and autism spectrum disorder: links and risks – a possible new overlap syndrome. *Pediatric Health, Medicine and Therapeutics, 6*, 153-166

[4] Horvath, K., Papadimitriou, J.C., Rabsztyn, A., Drachenberg, C., and Tildon, J.T. (1999). Gastrointestinal abnormalities in children with autistic disorder. *J Pediatr, 135*(5), 559-563

[5] Wasilewska, J. and Klukowski, M. (2015). Gastrointestinal symptoms and autism spectrum disorder: links and risks – a possible new overlap syndrome. *Pediatric Health, Medicine and Therapeutics, 6*, 153-166

[6] Feingold, S.M., Molitoris, D., Song, Y., Liu, C., Vaisanen, M.L., Bolte, E., ... Kaul, A. (2002) Gastrointestinal microflora studies in late-onset autism. *Clin Infect Dis, 35*(Suppl 1), S6-S16.

[7] Vojdani, A., Campbell, A.W., Anyanwu, E., Kashanian, A., Bock, K., and Vojdani, E. Antibodies to neuron-specific antigens in children with autism: possible cross-reaction with encephalitogenic proteins from milk, Chlamydia pneumonia and Streptococcus group A. *J Neuroimmunol, 129*(1-2), 168-177.

[8] Lucarelli, S., Fredlani, T., Zingoni, A.M., Ferruzzi, F., Giardini, O., Quinteri, F., ... Cardi, E. (1995). Food allergy and infantile autism. *Panminerva Med, 37*(3), 137-141.

[9] Knivsberg, A.M., Reichelt, K.L., Høien, T., and Nødland, M. (2013). A randomized, controlled study of dietary intervention in autistic syndrome. *Nutri Neurosci, 5*(4), 251-261

[10] Vojdani, A., Campbell, A.W., Anyanwu, E., Kashanian, A., Bock, K., and Vojdani, E. Antibodies to neuron-specific antigens in children with autism: possible cross-reaction with encephalitogenic proteins from milk, Chlamydia pneumonia and Streptococcus group A. *J Neuroimmunol, 129*(1-2), 168-177.

[11] Lucarelli, S., Fredlani, T., Zingoni, A.M., Ferruzzi, F., Giardini, O., Quinteri, F., ... Cardi, E. (1995). Food allergy and infantile autism. *Panminerva Med, 37*(3), 137-141.

[12] O'Banion, D., Armstrong, B., Cummings, R.A., and Stange, J. (1978). "Disruptive behavior: a dietary approach." *J Autism Child Schizophr, 8*(3), 325-337.

[13] Vojdani, A., O'Bryan, T., Green, J.A., Mccandless, J., Woeller, K.N., Vojdani, E., and Cooper, E.L. (2004). Immune response to dietary proteins, gliadin and cerebellar peptides in children with autism. *Nutr Neuroscience, 7*(3), 151-161.

[14] Kinney, H.C., Burger, P.C., Hurwitz, B.J., Hijmans, J.C., and Grant, J.P. (1982).

Degeneration of the central nervous system associated with celiac disease. *J Neurol Sci*, 53(1), 9-22

[15] DeSantis, A., Addolorato, G., Romito, A., Caputo, S., Giordano, A., Gambassi, G., ... Gasbarrini, G. (1997) Schizophrenia symptoms and SPECT abnormalities in a coelic patient: regression after luten-free diet. J Intern Med, 242(5). 421-423

[16] Beyenburg, S., Scheid, B., Deckert-Schluter, M., and Lagreze, H.L. (1998). Chronic progressive leukoencephalopathy in adult celiac disease. *Neurology*, 50(3), 820-822.

[17] Burk, K., Bosch, C.A., Melms, A., Zuhlke, C., Stern, M., Besenthal, I., ... Dichgans, J. (2001) Sporadic cerebellar ataxia associated with gluten sensitivity. Brain, 124(5), 1013-1019

[18] Hu, W.T., Murray, J.A., Greenaway, M.C., Parisi, J.E., and Josephs, K.A. (2006). Cognitive impairment and celiac disease. Arch Neurol, 63(10), 1440-1446

[19] Harvard Medical School. (2015, August 12). *The Autism-GI Link*. Retrieved from www.hms.harvard.edu/news/autism-gi-link

[20] Angelidou, A., Alysandratos, K.D., Asadi, S., Zhang, B., Francis, K., Vasiadi, M., ... Theoharides, T.C. (2011) Brief report: "allergic symptoms" in children with Autism Spectrum Disorders. More than meets the eye?. *J Autism Dev Disord*, 41(11), 1579-1585.

[21] Theoharides, T.C., Angelidou, A., Alysandratos, K.D., Zhang, B., Asadi, S., Francis, K., ... Kalogeromitros, D. (2012) Mast cell activation and autism. *Biochim Biophys Acta*, 1822(1), 34-41.

[22] Kempuraj, D., Asadi, S., Zhang, B., Manola, A., Hogan, J., Peterson, E., & Theoharides, T. C. (2010). Mercury induces inflammatory mediator release from human mast cells. *Journal of neuroinflammation*, 7, 20. doi:10.1186/1742-2094-7-20

[23] Theoharides, T.C., Stewart, J.M., Panagiotidou, S., and Melamed, I. (2016). Mast cells, brain inflammation and autism. *Eur J Pharmacol*, 778, 96-102.

[24] Theoharides, T.C., and Zhang, B. (2011). Neuro-Inflammation, Blood-Brain Barrier, Seizures and Autism. *Journal of Neuroinflammation*, 8, 168.

[25] Martínez-Martínez, L.A., Mora, T., Vargas, A., Fuentes-Iniestra, M., and Martínez-Lavín, M. (2014). Sympathetic nervous system dysfunction in fibromyalgia, chronic fatigue syndrome, irritable bowel syndrome, and interstitial cystitis: a review of case-control studies. *J Clin Rheumatol*, 20(3),

[26] Crawley, E., Hunt, L., and Stallard, P. (2009). Anxiety in children with CFS/ME. *Eur Child Adolesc Psychiatry*, 18(11), 683–689.

[27] Perricone, C., Colafrancesco, S., Mazor, R.D., Soriano, A., Agmon-Levin, N., and Shoenfeld, Y. (2013). Autoimmune/inflammatory syndrome induced by adjuvants (ASIA) 2013: Unveiling the pathogenic, clinical and diagnostic aspects. *Journal of Autoimmunity*, 47, 1-16.

[28] Watad, A., David, P., Brown, S., & Shoenfeld, Y. (2017). Autoimmune/Inflammatory Syndrome Induced by Adjuvants and Thyroid Autoimmunity. *Frontiers in endocrinology*, 7, 150. doi:10.3389/fendo.2016.00150

[29] Khan, Z., Combadière, C., Authier, F., Itier, V., Lux, F., Exley, C., …
Cadusseau, J. (2013). Slow CCL2-dependent translocation of biopersistent
particles from muscle to brain. *BMC Medicine*, 11, 99
[30] Shoenfield, Y., Agmon-Levin, N., and Tomljenovic, L. (Eds.). (2015) *Vaccines
and Autoimmunity* (1st edition, p.19). Hoboken, New Jersey: Wiley-Blackwell

CHAPTER 45

Alzheimer's and aluminum

*"Memory is all we are. Moments and
feelings, captured in amber, strung on filaments
of reason. Take a man's memories and you take
all of him. Chip away a memory at a time and
you destroy him as surely as if you hammered
nail after nail through his skull."*

~**Mark Lawrence** *(King of Thorns)*

We would also like to touch on the subject of Alzheimer's disease (AD) even though this does not affect children. We do believe it has some correlation to childhood diseases. The common denominator appears to be aluminum (Al) and other metals.

As you may recall, aluminum can be much more toxic once it's injected into the body. But as with so much else, we have to count on research that does not involve injections. Instead, we have to keep in mind the fact that being injected may potentially have greater adverse effects than what was observed in the studies.

Authors of one such study published in 2009 explain that we are exposed to aluminum "through air, food and water." They connect damage by free radicals and changes in neurological behavior to the impact aluminum has on the brain.

The authors also explain:

> *"However, there is no known physiological role for aluminium within the body and hence this metal may produce adverse physiological effects. Chronic exposure of animals to aluminium is associated with behavioural,*

325

neuropathological and neurochemical changes. Among them, deficits of learning and behavioural functions are most evident."[1]

Authors of a paper published in 2014, explain:

"[...] Alzheimer's disease is a manifestation of chronic Al neurotoxicity in humans. Because Al is similar to iron, it gains access to iron-dependent cells involved in memory." [2]

The authors continue by explaining that:

"[...] Al in human beings implicates Al toxicants as causally involved in Lou Gehrig's disease (ALS), Alzheimer's disease and autism spectrum disorders."[3]

This sparked a question in our minds: Is Alzheimer's disease (AD) the same as autism?

It appears to us that the difference between the two is with autism, everything happens a lot faster, while AD is a slower process and therefore occurs later in life. We are not so naïve as to believe this is the only difference. We are just curious whether there could be something to it.

Brain struggles

The incidence of autism around the globe is exploding. In 2014, an estimated 1% of the world's population had autism. That means more than 70,000,000 human beings were, and many no doubt still are, struggling to function with a damaged brain as a consequence of this disease.

The reports in from individual countries indicate the alarming scope of the problem.

According to the World Health Organization's (WHO) an announcement posted April 2017 on its website states: "[i]t is estimated that worldwide 1 in 160 children has an ASD."[4] Our concern with gathering worldwide data into one statistic is the fact that we don't know the various methodologies used for each country. In US alone, there are three different survey methods used (mentioned below) and they all derive data differently.

That being said, we would still like to see what the ASD prevalence data is in countries other than the US. The website *Focus for Health* has posted autism diagnosis for 18 different countries, including US with data from 2015, which shows one in 45 children with autism.

The website derived their data from each individual country and they link references to each. The most recent data is from Germany, Ireland, Hong Kong and Singapore from 2016 and 2017. Here it shows Germany with one in 263 children with autism diagnoses, Singapore with one in 149, Ireland with one in 65 and Hong Kong with one in 27.[5]

In November 2015 the National Health Statistics Reports released by the US Department of Health and Human Services published a questionnaire to assess whether the autism spike was a true incidence spike. They have been conducting National Health Interview Surveys (NHIS) since 1997, which include:

> *"[...] questions to determine the prevalence of children ever diagnosed with the developmental disabilities of ASD, intellectual disability (ID), and any other developmental delay (other DD)."*[6]

This questionnaire remained unchanged until 2014 when NHIS made some adjustment by adding more detailed analysis of ASD. In their report they show two other survey systems: Autism and Developmental Disabilities Monitoring Network (ADDM), and National Survey of Children's Health (NSCH). The researchers feel strongly about the NHIS's approach being the best of the three:

> *"NHIS represents the most in-depth health survey, with more than 12,000 sample-child interviews completed annually about health conditions, functional limitations, and health care access and utilizations. In-person interviews and strong response rates make NHIS the principal source of information on health of the noninstitutionalized population of the United States."*[7]

It's difficult to compare the three systems as they vary so much in the way they collect data. As described in the above quote, the NHIS surveys more than 12,000 children age three to 17 annually. The survey published in 2015 showed that "22.4 per 1,000 children" were diagnosed with ASD. That's 2.4% of all children in US age three to 17.

This may not seem like a high percentage, but let's say you have 5,000 children in your school district, 112 of them would have autism.

The reports show that in 2014 the autism rate nearly doubled from what it was from 2011–2013. As mentioned above, they contributed this to the more detailed description of ASD (i.e. inclusion of Asperger's disorder). Nonetheless, it doesn't explain the worldwide statistics.

The Survey shown for ADDM is from 2010 and covers 360,000 eight-year-old children. The data was collected by "[e]xpert clinicians review medical and education records and apply surveillance case definition"[8]. This survey showed an ASD prevalence of "14.7 per 1,000 children." The difference here is the data was collected from health professionals and therefore included children not officially diagnosed with ASD (~20% of survey subjects). Both NHIS and ADDM were funded by the CDC.

The last survey mentioned is the National Survey of Children's Health (NSCH) conducted by phone in 2011–2012. It highlighted "[p]aren't-reported survey responses about current autism spectrum disorder diagnosis." NSCH reached over 95,000 children aged six to 17 throughout the US. According to their data set, the autism prevalence in this age group was "20,0 per 1,000 children." This survey was funded by Human Resources & Services Administration (HRSA).[9]

More recent data from NSCH was published in the journal *Pediatrics* in November 2018. Using the same methods as described above, this study reached the carers of 43,283 children aged between three and 17. It showed by 2016 there was an ASD prevalence of "2.50 per 100 children" This means that an "estimated prevalence of US children with parent-reported ASD diagnosis is now 1 in 40"[10].

According to the CDC's website, ADDM data revealed one in 59 children had been diagnosed with autism by 2014.[11] With the steady increase in autism each year, NSCH's new data showing one in 40 children are being diagnosed with autism today doesn't seem so far-fetched.

Regardless, it's safe to say that ASD is on the rise and becoming more prevalent than ever before.

Another disease that perhaps not many have heard of is Pink Acrodonia, often referred to as *the Pink disease*. Caused by mercury in teething powder, this disease seems to have disappeared after the 1950s. The reason we mention Pink Acrodonia is because it has all the hallmarks and behaviors of an autistic child from head banging to a disconnect with other people.

A study was done on the grandchildren of those who survived pink disease to see if there were genetic factors involved. They found that one out 22 pink disease survivors had grandchildren with ASD, while one out 160 from the general population had grandchildren with ASD.[12]

Other than autism

We also found a paper that looks at the causal effect between vaccines, the immune system and brain development. The authors of that study appear to feel vaccines are important and do not seem to support the link between MMR and autism. They state directly that "this association has been convincingly disproven." Even so, they feel there are other disorders worth a second look. These include obsessive-compulsive disorder (OCD, anorexia nervosa (AN), "tic disorder, anxiety disorder, ADHD, major depressive disorder, and bipolar disorder."[13]

The study looks at correlation between these disorders and various vaccines. Among these vaccines were vaccines for "tetanus and diphtheria (TD), hepatitis A, hepatitis B, meningitis, and varicella."

At the end of paper, they state:

> "[...] preliminary epidemiologic evidence that the onset of some pediatric-onset neuropsychiatric disorders, including AN, OCD, anxiety disorders, and tic disorders, may be temporally related to prior vaccinations."[14]

The authors also stress that this is not proof of causal relationship. Whether they and others of the same viewpoint are right or wrong, the results from the study done on grandchildren of pink disease victims could hold the underlying answer.

Our body has an innate ability to edit its DNA codes. This also means that when it is exposed to toxins, the editing process can be distorted and cause errors which become imbedded into the DNA. These errors are then passed on to offspring and render them more susceptible to toxic injuries or other disadvantages the errors may cause.

The connection between the pink disease and autism brings to the fore something that has been brewing in the back of our minds for a while. It's something we haven't addressed yet, but feel strongly it deserves at least a passing mention before we end this book. We refer to the topic covered in the next and our last chapter: DNA epigenetics.

Chapter 45: Alzheimer's and aluminum

[1] Kumar, V. and Gill, K.D. (2009). Aluminium neurotoxicity: neurobehavioural and oxidative aspects. *Arch Toxicol*, 83(11), 965-978.

[2] Shaw, C., Seneff, S., Kette, S.D., Tomljenovic, L., Oller Jr. J.W., and Davidson, R.M. (2014). Aluminum-Induced Entropy in Biological Systems: Implications for Neurological Disease. *Journal of Toxicology*, 2014, 491316

[3] Ibid.

[4] World Health Organization. (2017, April 4). *Autism spectrum disorders*. Retrieved from www.who.int/en/news-room/fact-sheets/detail/autism-spectrum-disorders

[5] Focus for Health (2017, August 28). *Autism Rates across the Developed World*. Retrieved from www.focusforhealth.org/autism-rates-across-the-developed-world/

[6] Zablotsky, B., Black, L.I, Maenner, M.J., Schieve, L.A., and Blumberg, S.J. (2015). Estimated Prevalence of Autism and Other Developmental Disabilities Following Questionnaire Changes in the 2014 National Health Interview Survey. *National Health Statistics Report*, 87, 1-20

[7] Ibid.

[8] Ibid.

[9] Ibid.

[10] Kogan, M.D., Vladutiu, C.J., Schieve, L.A., Ghandour, R.M., Blumberg, S.J., Zablotsky, B., … Lu, M.C. (2018). The Prevalence of Parent-Reported Autism Spectrum Disorder Among US Children. *Pediatrics*, 142(6)

[11] Centers for Disease Control and Prevention. (2018, November 15). *Autism Spectrum Disorder (ACD)*. Retrieved from www.cdc.gov/ncbddd/autism/data.html

[12] Shandley, K., & Austin, D. W. (2011). Ancestry of pink disease (infantile acrodynia) identified as a risk factor for autism spectrum disorders. *Journal of toxicology and environmental health. Part A*, 74(18), 1185-1194.

[13] Leslie, D. L., Kobre, R. A., Richmand, B. J., Aktan Guloksuz, S., & Leckman, J. F. (2017). Temporal Association of Certain Neuropsychiatric Disorders Following Vaccination of Children and Adolescents: A Pilot Case-Control Study. *Frontiers in psychiatry*, 8, 3. doi:10.3389/fpsyt.2017.00003

[14] Ibid.

CHAPTER 46

Our final word on vaccines

"Learn from yesterday, live for today, hope for tomorrow. The important thing is not to stop questioning."

~ **Albert Einstein** *(Theoretical physicist)*

The ongoing discussion on the association between vaccines and our natural immune responses appears to be, in some cases, all over the place. It's nearly, if not entirely, impossible to argue a definitive case in this matter.

But to continue on where we left off, let's delve right into epigenetics.

What science tells us is that who we are is written in our DNA, which means we have already been coded for what we are before we are even born. As we didn't have the opportunity to choose the DNA we are made of, it seems we can blame our genes for our mishaps. After all, we were born this way and there's nothing we can do about it.

But how do we explain the *placebo effect* whether it be as a biproduct of the environment (i.e. positive/negative reinforcement) or in the form of medication? Does it benefit us to blame our DNA since we have no power over it?

If genes are the main controlling factor, then why do we humans have about the same amount of genes as mice or dogs? Not only that, vegetables and wheat far exceed humans in the number of genes in their genome.

It's a conundrum to us how much simpler lifeforms have far more genes than us, especially if our genes are so important to who we become.

This also brings up something we mentioned earlier in the book. When scientists are making vaccines, what are some of the things they have to consider? You guessed it, environmental factors. They have to take into account such things as temperature, nutrition, pH balance, etc. What happens if these factors are not taken into account? The germ doesn't grow.

But, let's stop for a second. What has changed in the germ?

Bacterium is a single cell organism. The virus has mechanisms that are designed to replicate when in contact with a cell. Once the bacteria or virus are in the laboratory, do they automatically change what they are made of?

Our hypothesis is that the environment, be it in form of thoughts, living conditions, nutritional intake or medication, not to mention whatever factors are introduced to our cells, may all play a part in the make up of our DNA. If the environment doesn't accommodate the germ's basic survival mechanisms, it will simply just stop functioning properly or die. So, this means that environmental factors play a part in dictating to our genes, right?

Then are our genes set in stone? Can we actually alter our genes by changing environmental factors?

If you look at it this way, at the very core, our DNA structure is dictated to by atoms (carbon, hydrogen, oxygen, nitrogen, phosphorus). This means that DNA is electrically charged. It would only be natural that the atoms would be affected by electrical impulses in their environment. We won't go any further into this slightly philosophical epigenetic discussion, but while keeping in mind the environment, like us, is made up of atoms, we'll skip right into how epigenetics can affect the physical structure of DNA.

Our understanding and hypothesis, is that the environment, whether it be in form of thoughts, living conditions, nutritional intake, medication, and whatever factors that are introduced to our cells, may play a part in what happens. If these factors don't benefit the cell, the cell won't adjust to function properly.

These thoughts about epigenetics didn't come to us out of thin air. We have the remarkable zoologist, Jean-Baptiste Lamarck (1744–1829) to thank. While some of his theories may have been discredited, many are still incredibly fascinating and thought-provoking. Even Charles Darwin acknowledged him as "justly-celebrated naturalist."[1]

A quote from Lamarck that sparked this way of thinking in us was:

> *"It is not the organs — that is, the character and form of the animal's bodily parts — that have given rise to its habits and particular structures. It is the habits and manner of life and the conditions in which its ancestors lived that have in the course of time fashioned its bodily form, its organs and qualities."*[2]

Delving into DNA epigenetics means we are no longer just dealing with gene mutations, but also switching the genes on or off (referred to briefly in previous chapter). On our DNA we have something called Methylation variable positions (MVP), which are epigenetics markers. In order to alter the function of the DNA, a methyl (CH_3) group is added to the DNA. This is called methylation.

When methylation takes place, it happens at the CpG sequence site. The CpG sequence is simply when the nucleotides cytosine (C) and guanine (G) are next to each other in the DNA sequence. In between each nucleotide is phosphate (p) that holds them together. Hence CpG. It is at this sequence we see methylation. The CpG sequences make sure the genes are being expressed correctly.

When the MVP (which is located at the CpG site) is altered, an epigenetic pattern is created. This can affect the cell at any time during cell maturation. This goes for cancer cells as well. Among the substances able to affect this pattern are toxins and germs. When DNA methylation has taken place, the alteration tends to stay around even after cell division. This way the new epigenetic pattern may potentially become a part of a new cell population.

An example of how this can affect generations can be seen in a 2006 paper not related to vaccines.

The authors of that paper say that where:

> *"[...] epigenetic variation whereby the environment induces stable phenotypic changes without any genetic changes. [...]. That is, the individual, with its adapted morphological, physiological and behavioral traits, can be both a result and a cause of evolutionary change."*[3]

We don't want to get into a lengthy discussion on epigenetics so we will leave this subject by quoting from another paper published in 2007:

"The ability of environmental factors to influence evolutionary processes has led to the speculation that epigenetic mechanisms are a significant determinant factor in evolution. A combination of DNA sequence mutation (i.e., classic genetic processes) and epigenetic processes are postulated to be important for evolutionary adaptation events."[4]

So, what exactly does our DNA do? It codes for all our physical and emotional traits? A grand study was published in 2016 to find correlation between our genes and personality traits.[5] Not only did the study find genes that correlated with personality traits, but were also able to correlate a location on our genes to illnesses such as attention-deficit/hyperactivity disorder (ADHD) and depression/anxiety. They made sure to mention that environmental factors also play a role.

Viruses are a most fascinating phenomenon. Some say that viruses are not living, but we say that some vaccines are *live* viral vaccines. You may ask how can a non-living thing be alive in a vaccine? Viruses are not alive in the sense that they don't have the internal machinery of a normal cell. They are not an active, intelligent entity, but rather exist in a passive manner. It seems to be more about whether the virus is harmful or not.

Viruses don't just float around and infect. Instead, they enter the human body, and use the human cellular ingredients for their own benefit. One can therefore say that a virus is just as much a part of humans as they are of themselves. They cannot infect us without using human cells to participate in the process.

A virus needs a living cell to multiply and will spend its lifetime finding a place where it can grow. If we vaccinate against a virus, another virus will step into the void in its stead. It may seem like the virus finds us and infects us, even kills us, but the case for them is merely happenstance. Viruses happen to be in an environment that allows them to replicate, and so they do. There's no intelligence or order behind this, it simply comes down to the fact that the right mechanisms are in place for it to happen.

At first, it may seem that it's all about the virus and what we need to do to protect ourselves against it or other specific viruses. In the meantime, we forget it is first and foremost all about us. Without us, the virus cannot replicate.

The same goes for other germs. It's all about the environment we prepare for them. Will we offer them a welcoming environment where they can thrive and take over? Or do we focus first and foremost on how to keep our cells healthy and thereby provide an uninviting place for any parasitic relationship to develop?

There's a theory that the virus needs the host insomuch as, when allowed to stay, it will actually cause the host less harm. When we constantly create vaccines against certain strains or diseases, these germs, in return, will find a mutated and often more virulent way to survive in order to remain in the host.

With this in mind, let's not forget that many of these germs have co-evolved side by side

with us throughout history. These have often turned out to be beneficial to our health and also necessary for our survival.

Viruses find their way into our bodies. Once inside, they rewrite parts of our DNA. This has been happening for a very long time. We as humans have been able to take advantage of this mutualistic relationship with viruses. A relationship that is also commensalistic in that one organism receives a benefit, or benefits, from the other while the other one's not affected. For example, our placenta has retroviral DNA. Without it, we would not be able to have a functioning placenta.

Are we messing with a necessary evolutionary process by changing the wild strains into mutated strains and/or vaccine strains? Have we created enemies out of what used to be, for the most part, our friends?

Germs have been strengthening our immune system throughout human history. It wasn't until relatively recently we started injecting ourselves with substances to prevent them from doing *their job*.

This is a brand-new way of dealing with incoming unknowns that don't fit the way our immune system evolved. And this new method is bypassing a system as old as Mankind, so we have to expect there will be some kind of adverse reaction.

We can't help but wonder if we keep introducing antigens to our bodies in this manner, where will this new evolutionary path take us? And will vaccinations, and the modern immunization process in general, ultimately be classified as a transhumanist methodology? Transhumanist in that this experimental approach is attempting to use science and technology to evolve the human race beyond its current physical limitations or weaknesses, which is after all the definition of transhumanism.

They say keep your friends close, but your enemies closer. What if the germs are the enemy? How close should we keep them?

Well, germs have been strengthening our immune system throughout human history. (Hopefully, we've successfully gotten that message across by now). It wasn't until relatively recently we started injecting ourselves with substances to prevent germs from doing their job.

Vaccinations are, in evolutionary terms at least, a brand new way of dealing with incoming unknowns that don't fit the way our immune system evolved. And this new methodology is bypassing a system as old as Mankind itself, so we have to expect there will be adverse reactions of some kind from time to time.

We cannot help but wonder...

If we keep introducing antigens to our bodies in this manner, where will this new evolutionary path take us?

Chapter 46: Our final word on vaccines

[1] Darwin, C.R. (c1909). *The Origin of Species.* (p.10). New York, U.S.A.: P.F. Collier

[2] Asimov, I. (1988). *Book of Science and Nature Quotations – Isaac Asimov.* (p.215). Asimov, I. and Shulman, J.A. (Eds.). New York, U.S.A.: Weidenfeld & Nicolson.

[3] Crews, D. and McLachlan, J.A. (2006). Epigenetics, Evolution, Endocrine Disruption, Health, and Disease. *Endocrinology,* 147(6 Suppl), S4-10

[4] Crews, D., Gore, A. C., Hsu, T. S., Dangleben, N. L., Spinetta, M., Schallert, T., Anway, M. D., ... Skinner, M. K. (2007). Transgenerational epigenetic imprints on mate preference. *Proceedings of the National Academy of Sciences of the United States of America,* 104(14), 5942-5946.

[5] Lo, M-T., Hinds, D.A., Tung, J.Y., Franz, C., Fan, C-C., Wang, Y., ... Chen, C-H. (2016). Genome-wide analyses for personality traits identify six genomic loci and show correlations with psychiatric disorders. *Nature Genetics,* 49, 152-156 (2017).

Vaccine overview

Table includes ingredients discussed in this book. For a more comprehensive list, please refer to package inserts or other reliable internet sources.

Vaccine	Type	Name	Manuf.
HepA	Inactivated virus	Havrix[1]	GSK
HepA	Inactivated virus	Vaqta[2]	Merck
Polio	Inactivated virus	IPOL[3]	Sanofi Pasteur
MMR	Live virus	MMR II[4]	Merck
MMR	Live virus	ProQuad[5]	Merck
Rotavirus	Live virus oral	Rotarix[6]	GSK
Rotavirus	Live virus oral	RotaTeq[7]	Merck
Varicella	Live virus	Varivax[8]	Merck
HepB	Gen. Engineered	Engerix-B[9]	GSK
HepB	Gen. Engineered	Recombivax[10]	Merck
DTaP	Toxoid Subunit	Daptacel[11]	Sanofi Pasteur
DTaP	Toxoid Subunit	Infanrix[12]	GSK
Pneumococcal	Polysac. Subunit	Prevnar 13[13]	Pfizer
Meningococcal	Polysac. Subunit	Menactra[14]	Sanofi P
Meningococcal	Oligosac. Subunit	Menveo[15]	Novartis
Hib	Polysac. subunit	ActHIB[16]	Sanofi Pasteur
Hib	Polysac. subunit	Hiberix[17]	GSK
Hib	Polysac. subunit	PedvaxHIB[18]	Merck

Vaccine	Additional DNA	Other
HepA	MRC-5	Al., F., P20, neomycin
	MRC-5, bovine	Al., F., neomycin
Polio	Vero cells, bovine	F, neomycin, polymyxin b, streptomycin, P80
MMR	Chick embryo, WI-38, bovine	MSG, gelatin, neomycin
MMR	Chick embryo, WI-38, MRC-5, bovine	MSG, gelatin, neomycin
Rotavirus	Vero cells, PCV1, bovine	
	Vero cells, PCV1&2, bovine	P80
Varicella	MRC-5, WI-38, guinea pig, bovine	MSG, gelatin, neomycin
HepB	Yeast	Al
	Yeast	Al., F.
DTaP	Bovine	Al., F
	Bovine	Al., F., P80
Pneumococcal	Soy, Yeast, bovine, diptheria CRM	Al., P80
Meningococcal	Bovine, diptheria	F
	Diptheria CRM, yeast	F
Hib	Tetanus toxoid, bovine,	F
	Tetanus toxoid,	F
	N.meningitidis,	Al.

Appendix 1: Vaccine overview

[1] Glaxo Smith Kline. (2016, May). *Havrix*. Retrieved from www.gsksource.com/pharma/content/dam/GlaxoSmithKline/US/en/Prescribing_Information/Havrix/pdf/HAVRIX.PDF

[2] Merck. (2014, February). *Vaqta*. Retrieved from www.merck.com/product/usa/pi_circulars/v/vaqta/vaqta_pi.pdf

[3] Sanofi. (2008, August 21). *IPOL*. Retrieved from www.products.sanofi.com.au/vaccines/IPOL_NZ_PI.pdf

[4] Merck. (n.d.). *M-M-R II*. Retrieved from www.merck.com/product/usa/pi_circulars/m/mmr_ii/mmr_ii_pi.pdf

[5] Food and Drug Administration. (n.d.). *ProQuad*. Retrieved from www.fda.gov/downloads/biologicsbloodvaccines/vaccines/approvedproducts/ucm123796.pdf

[6] Glaxo Smith Kline. (2016, April). *Rotarix*. Retrieved from www.gsksource.com/pharma/content/dam/GlaxoSmithKline/US/en/Prescribing_Information/Rotarix/pdf/ROTARIX-PI-PIL.PDF

[7] Merck. (2018, March). *RotaTeq*. Retrieved from www.merck.com/product/usa/pi_circulars/r/rotateq/rotateq_pi.pdf

[8] Food and Drug Administration. (2018, October). *Varivax*. Retrieved from www.fda.gov/downloads/BiologicsBloodVaccines/Vaccines/ApprovedProducts/UCM142812.pdf

[9] Food and Drug Administration. (n.d.). *Engerix-B*. Retrieved from www.fda.gov/downloads/biologicsbloodvaccines/vaccines/approvedproducts/ucm224503.pdf

[10] Food and Drug Administration. (n.d.). *Recombivax HB*. Retrieved from www.fda.gov/downloads/biologicsbloodvaccines/vaccines/approvedproducts/ucm110114.pdf

[11] Food and Drug Administration. (n.d.). *Daptacel*. Retrieved from www.fda.gov/downloads/biologicsbloodvaccines/vaccines/approvedproducts/ucm103037.pdf

[12] Food and Drug Administration. (n.d.). *Infanrix*. Retrieved from www.fda.gov/downloads/biologicsbloodvaccines/vaccines/approvedproducts/ucm124514.pdf

[13] Food and Drug Administration. (2018, April). *Menactra*. Retrieved from www.fda.gov/downloads/BiologicsBloodVaccines/Vaccines/ApprovedProducts/UCM574852.pdf

[14] Food and Drug Administration. (2018, August). *Prevnar 13*. Retrieved from www.fda.gov/downloads/biologicsbloodvaccines/vaccines/approvedproducts/ucm131170.pdf

[15] Food and Drug Administration. (n.d.). *Menveo*. Retrieved from www.fda.gov/downloads/biologicsbloodvaccines/vaccines/approvedproducts/ucm201349.pdf

[16] Food and Drug Administration. (n.d.). *ActHib*. Retrieved from www.fda.gov/downloads/biologicsbloodvaccines/vaccines/approvedproducts/ucm109841.pdf

[17] Food and Drug Administration. (2018, April). *Hiberix*. Retrieved from www.fda.gov/downloads/biologicsbloodvaccines/vaccines/approvedproducts/ucm179530.pdf

[18] Merck. (2018, May). Liquid PedvaxHIB. Retrieved from www.merck.com/product/usa/pi_circulars/p/pedvax_hib/pedvax_pi.pdf

OTHER BOOKS BY LANCE & JAMES MORCAN

published by Sterling Gate Books

Historical Fiction:

White Spirit (A novel based on a true story)
Into the Americas (A novel based on a true story)
World Odyssey (The World Duology, #1)
Fiji: A Novel (The World Duology, #2)

Conspiracy Thrillers:

The Ninth Orphan (The Orphan Trilogy, #1)
The Orphan Factory (The Orphan Trilogy, #2)
The Orphan Uprising (The Orphan Trilogy, #3)

Crime Thrillers:

Silent Fear (A novel inspired by true crimes)
The Heathrow Affair
The Me Too Girl

Action-Adventure:

The Dogon Initiative
High Country Contract

Non-Fiction:

DEBUNKING HOLOCAUST DENIAL THEORIES:
Two Non-Jews Affirm the Historicity of the Nazi Genocide

THE ORPHAN CONSPIRACIES:
29 Conspiracy Theories from The Orphan Trilogy

GENIUS INTELLIGENCE:
Secret Techniques and Technologies to Increase IQ
(The Underground Knowledge Series, #1)

ANTIGRAVITY PROPULSION:
Human or Alien Technologies?
(The Underground Knowledge Series, #2)

MEDICAL INDUSTRIAL COMPLEX:
The $ickness Industry, Big Pharma and Suppressed Cures
(The Underground Knowledge Series, #3)

THE CATCHER IN THE RYE ENIGMA:
J.D. Salinger's Mind Control Triggering Device or a Coincidental
Literary Obsession of Criminals?
(The Underground Knowledge Series, #4)

INTERNATIONAL BANKSTER$:
The Global Banking Elite Exposed and the Case for Restructuring
Capitalism
(The Underground Knowledge Series, #5)

BANKRUPTING THE THIRD WORLD:
How the Global Elite Drown Poor Nations in a Sea of Debt
(The Underground Knowledge Series, #6)

UNDERGROUND BASES:
Subterranean Military Facilities and the Cities Beneath Our Feet
(The Underground Knowledge Series, #7)

Short Stories by Lance Morcan

5 SHORT STORY GEMS:
Once Were Brothers / Mr. 100% / A Gladiator's Love / The Last
Tasmanian Tiger / Brooklyn Bankster

www.ingramcontent.com/pod-product-compliance
Lightning Source LLC
Chambersburg PA
CBHW021918190326
41519CB00009B/824